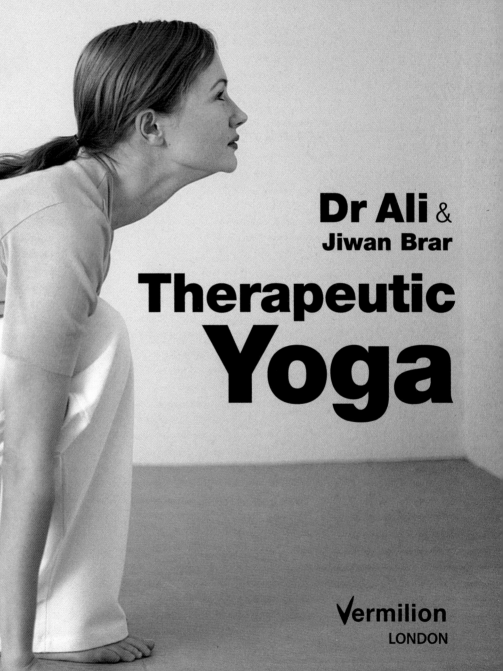

**Promote your body's
natural healing powers
with this revolutionary
approach to yoga**

Dr Ali &
Jiwan Brar

Therapeutic
Yoga

Vermilion

LONDON

For our parents

First published in Great Britain in 2002

1 3 5 7 9 10 8 6 4 2

Text © Dr Mosaraf Ali and Jiwan Brar 2002
Photographs © Winfried Heinze 2002

First published by Vermilion, an imprint of Ebury Press
Random House, 20 Vauxhall Bridge Road, London SW1V 2SA

Random House Australia (Pty) Limited
20 Alfred Street, Milsons Point, Sydney, New South Wales 2061, Australia

Random House New Zealand Limited
18 Poland Road, Glenfield, Auckland 10, New Zealand

Random House South Africa (Pty) Limited
Endulini, 5A Jubilee Road, Parktown 2193, South Africa

The Random House Group Limited
Reg. No. 954009

www.randomhouse.co.uk

A CIP catalogue record for this book is available from the British Library.

Editor Rachel Aris
Designers Maggie Town and Beverly Price
Photographer Winfried Heinze

ISBN 0091885140

Colour separation by Colorlito, Milan

Printed and bound in Singapore by Tien Wah Press

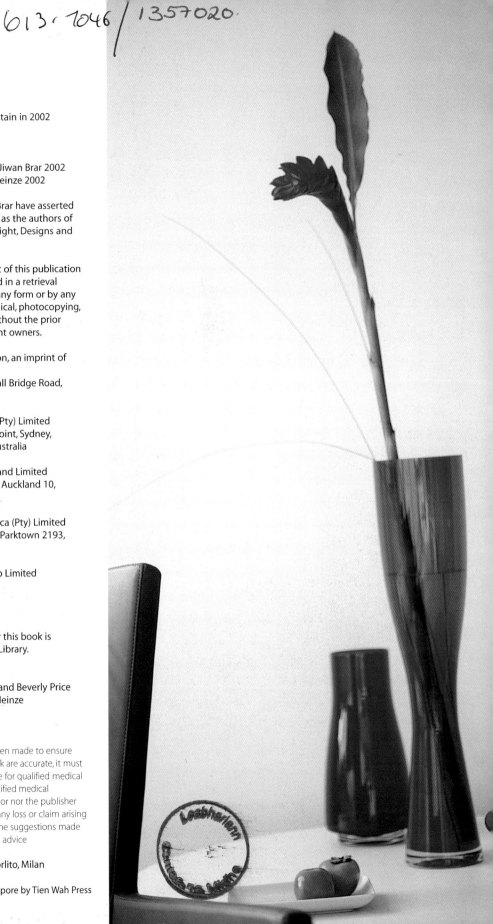

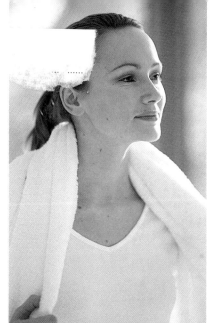

Therapeutic
Yoga

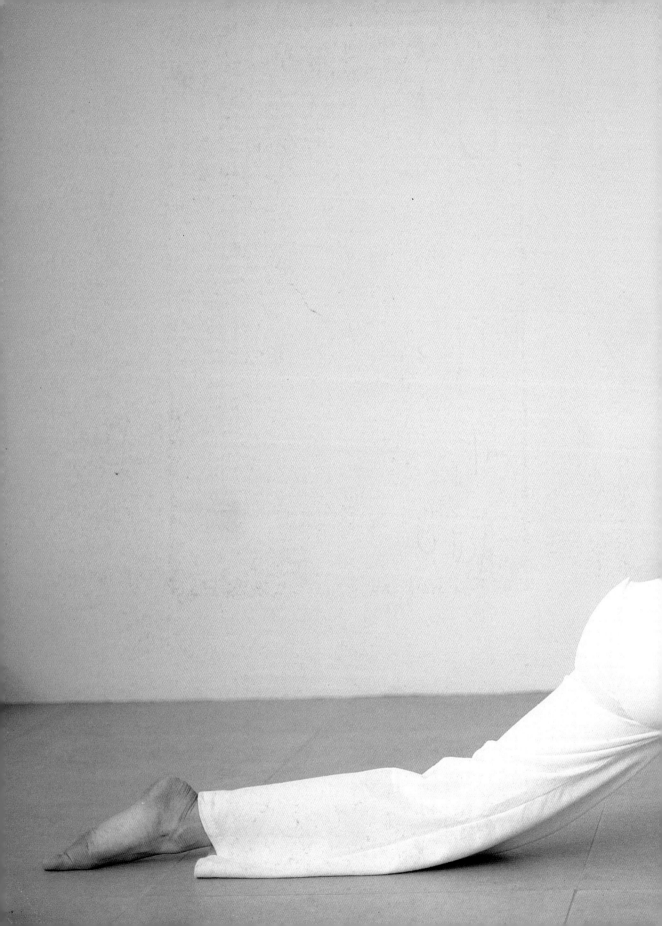

contents

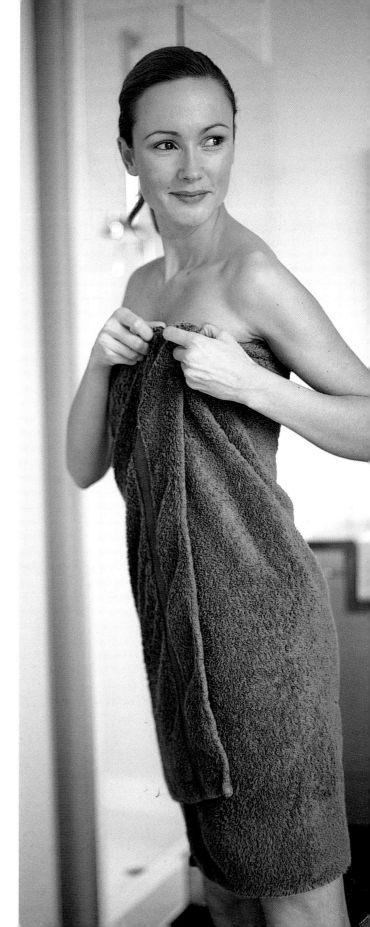

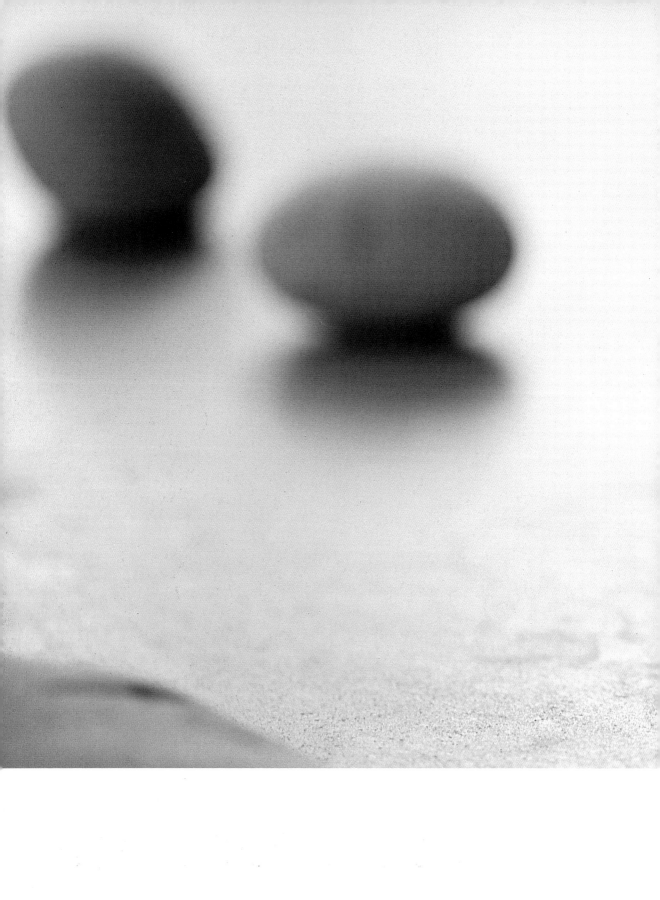

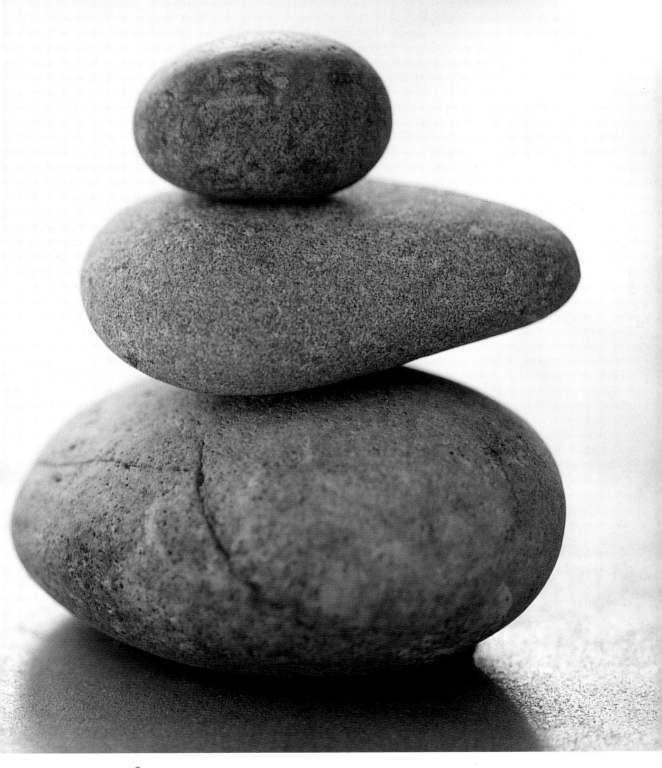

part 1
what is therapeutic yoga?

the tradition of yoga

Although yoga is relatively new to the West, it has a long and venerable tradition in the East. It is thought to date back to at least 3000 BC, and has been practised in India to promote physical and spiritual health for millennia. The first text on classical yoga, known as the *Yoga Sutras*, was written by a legendary yogi called Patanjali around 200 BC. Patanjali's path towards self-knowledge is known as Ashtanga or eight-limbed yoga, as it consists of eight steps to enlightenment. These steps help to discipline the body, mind, breath, emotions and spirit. Increasingly, we are realising that health no longer 'happens' at the physical level alone: for example, emotions can trigger the release of certain chemicals in the brain that may affect the body's long-term health. This is why yoga is so good for you: it promotes wellbeing at every level.

Yoga was originally popularised in the West during the 1960s by a number of gurus, spiritual leaders and philosophers who promoted all things Indian. Their approach to life appealed hugely to many rock stars and celebrities as it contrasted starkly with the materialistic approach that predominated in the West at the time. The search for alternative ways of life contributed to the growth of the hippy movement, and many people travelled to India to enjoy the slow, peaceful pace of life and follow the trail to true bliss. But with so many new experiences to explore – including free love, drugs and psychedelia – some of the finer aspects of Eastern culture, such as yoga, meditation and spirituality, were largely overlooked.

For a while, yoga and meditation remained a mystery to the West. Rather than being mainstream activities, they were taught by gurus who advocated strict discipline and a complete change in lifestyle; many teachers promoted vegetarianism – which was quite radical a few decades ago! Most people, however, couldn't see the point in twisting the body into strange configurations often named after an animal or object, and they were wary of levitation and other advanced stages of meditative practice. (In fact, there's nothing very mystical about levitation: the anti-gravitational force created by the spinal muscles stretching upwards makes it easy for someone who has mastered the art to spring up from a sitting position.)

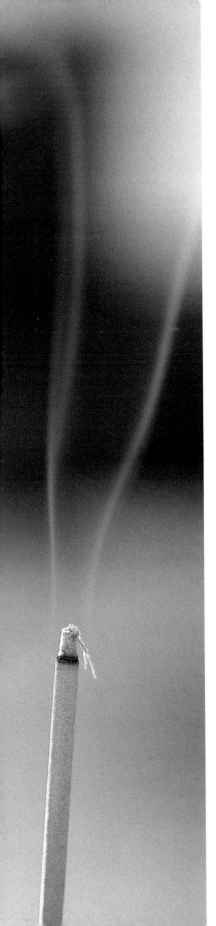

Some gurus used yoga simply as a tool to show off their skills and compete with each other. Yet in doing so, they went against the very principles of yoga – humility, tolerance, restraint, calm and detachment – and concentrated instead on the physical and aesthetic. The West thus interpreted yoga as a series of exercises and thought of it in much the same way as other forms of physical activities and gymnastics. What's more, many people worried it would take years to master the many complicated positions. But the fact is that yoga is a suitable form of exercise and relaxation for everyone, of all ages and abilities. Beginners aren't expected to perform the full postures straight away: modified versions are still very beneficial, and often essential if the practitioner is experiencing health problems.

Over the last decade or so, yogic exercise has become increasingly popular. Thanks to the efforts of some celebrities, together with the modern preoccupation with fitness and stress management, yoga has become a household name and is now an established form of physical exercise. Yet, in its original form, yoga is so much more than just a system of exercise. Traditionally, there are many different aspects of yoga, including karma yoga (the yoga of action, selfless service and charity), raja yoga (the science of physical and mental control), bhakti yoga (the yoga of love and devotion through prayer and worship) and jnana yoga (the yoga of knowledge and wisdom). Hatha, or therapeutic, yoga is part of raja yoga. Other types include yantra (visual) yoga, kundalini yoga (which stimulates the subconscious or the autonomic nervous system) and tantric yoga (in which the body is used to master the psychic processes).

For those in the know, yoga is not simply a series of poses but a whole way of life, encompassing diet, massage, relaxation and meditation. As well as being a great way to stay in shape, it also promotes the body's natural healing powers, and can be used by anyone to treat a wide range of health problems, both physical and emotional. This is the first book to explore fully the therapeutic effects of yoga.

the benefits of therapeutic yoga

The word 'yoga' comes from a Sanskrit word meaning 'union', and it symbolises the harmonisation of the body with the mind. Therapeutic yoga is a new name but an old concept. Known to the yoga masters for centuries, it is an all-inclusive therapy – involving breath control, physical movements or exercises (hatha yoga), massage or manipulative techniques, meditation and relaxation – which harnesses the body's natural healing powers, helping to boost your all-round wellbeing and to promote a speedier recovery when you do fall ill.

Part 2 of the book (pages 24–47) is devoted to a Healthy Living Routine aimed at keeping you in optimum health. This consists of advice on your everyday diet, how to massage yourself or a partner, breathing exercises, yoga poses that are suitable for regular practice, plus relaxation techniques. If you are able to incorporate this programme into your daily life, you will reap great rewards, including better health, more energy, improved concentration, less stress and a calmer state of mind.

We don't, however, live in an ideal world, and even if we practise yoga every day, our innate healing powers can be weakened by the stressful environments we live in. This is

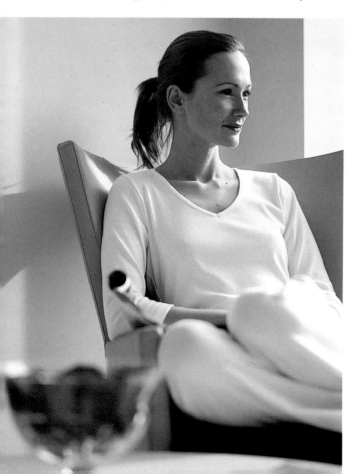

where therapeutic yoga comes in. Part 3 of the book (pages 48–141) looks at a variety of common ailments and explains how to use therapeutic yoga to eliminate or alleviate symptoms, as well as tackle the root cause of the problem. Here you will find recommendations for adapting your diet to treat each condition; special massage techniques to improve blood flow and help relieve discomfort; and a specially devised sequence of yoga postures, or asanas, for each different ailment – each posture having been carefully chosen, and in some cases adapted, for its specific healing powers. Repetitions have been suggested to adjust your body to these

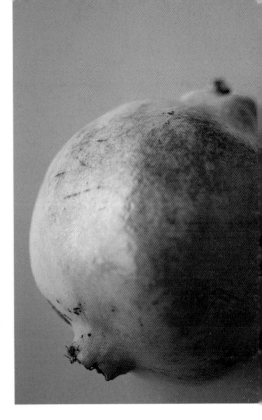

movements; but over time, the aim is to stay in the posture a little longer, and eventually you may need to repeat it just once but hold it for longer (12 breaths). This will make it easy to follow to bring about the desired therapeutic effect.

Each aspect of therapeutic yoga – diet, massage, the yoga postures, breath control and meditation – has specific benefits and is an important therapy in itself, but together they form a very powerful healing tool, as follows:

a healthy diet

According to yogic wisdom, nutritious eating is as important as regularly performing the asanas. A balanced diet will provide all the nutrients you need not only to keep physically fit but also to stay mentally sharp and in excellent health. The key to dietary wellbeing is variety and moderation. There is a huge range of fresh ingredients to choose from, which will help to support your physical and spiritual development. Certain foods, however, have deleterious effects on the digestive system. Our dietary advice therefore focuses mainly on foods to avoid. In Part 2 we have included details of ingredients to limit or cut out from your daily diet: see pages 26–27. But some foods are particularly harmful if you have specific health issues, so we have included dietary recommendations under each of the ailments covered in Part 3 of the book. You can find further useful advice on what, how and when to eat on pages 52–54.

healing massage

This forms an essential part of our treatment programme. Massage has always been a powerful type of therapy, and as far back as Greek and Roman times it was used not only for physical and emotional relaxation, but also to treat aches, pains and fatigue. Somehow, though, it fell out of fashion in Europe, and until recently it was considered merely as a method of relaxation or pampering. In the East, however, massage continued to play an important therapeutic role, and in India, Japan, China, Thailand and throughout most of Asia it has evolved into a variety of different techniques, some using pressure points (as in acupressure), others stretching the muscles and

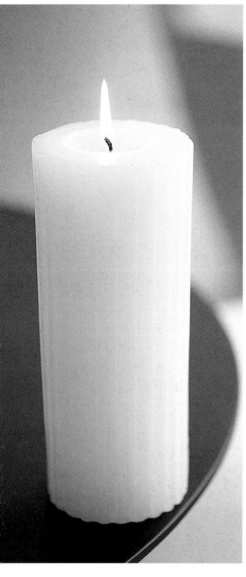

tendons, while others still use trigger points located deep within the muscles, nerve endings and joints. Massage has many benefits:

It removes the lactic acid that forms 'knots' within muscles Lactic acid builds up during periods of intense activity (it is produced when the body needs to burn lots of energy, for instance when you are sprinting, and the demand for oxygen in the muscles outstrips supply) and causes tightness, pain and fatigue. Massage can break down this lactic acid and reinvigorate the muscles.

It helps to overcome fatigue One of the main functions of blood circulation is that it supplies oxygen and nutrients to all the body tissues and removes toxins and by-products from them. When the muscles are squeezed during a massage, the waste products in the stagnant blood are expelled. Then, when they are released again, the muscles and the blood vessels gradually dilate and bring more blood in, with fresh oxygen and nutrients. As a result, the muscles function more efficiently. Because the muscles are responsible for producing most of the body's energy, more efficient muscles make for greater energy. Massage is particularly helpful, therefore, for treating energy-sapping disorders such as chronic fatigue syndrome (also known as ME or post-viral fatigue: see pages 107–108).

It relieves aches and pains in the joints The ligaments and tendons around joints have a poor blood supply, so when they are injured they heal very slowly and often become inflamed. Massage brings in more blood and helps to remove various by-products of the inflammatory process, thereby assisting the healing process.

It alleviates spinal problems Besides movement, the main function of the muscles in the spine and legs is to maintain correct posture. If these muscles are weakened or damaged, many painful disorders such as backache and osteoarthritis can develop. Massage of the postural muscles in the spine, legs and feet helps to keep these muscles in peak condition.

It activates the innate healing abilities of the body Much has been written about the healing power of touch, and there is no doubt in our minds that some kind of energy is passed on to the person receiving the massage from the person giving it. This boosts the body's energy and thus the subject's own recuperative potential.

An all-over, deep-tissue massage, if received on a regular basis, will help to invigorate your muscles and keep your body in good general condition. We have therefore included simple massage techniques in the Healthy Living Routine (see pages 28–31). But massage can also be employed more specifically as a therapeutic tool, and you will find suggestions in Part 3 of the book on how to use massage to treat particular conditions.

Therapeutic massage works in several different ways. Firstly, you can treat an area of the body that is directly affected by an injury or suffers from debilitating aches and pains. For example, if you sprain an ankle, massage the ligaments that have been injured shortly after the swelling goes down or the bruise appears. This helps to get the blood into the ligaments to provide nourishment for the inflammation to subside. After a few sessions of therapeutic massage, the ligaments will have healed and you can strengthen them again with suitable exercises. You can also use therapeutic massage in this way during an attack of tonsillitis. By massaging the lymph nodes in the neck, you encourage the lymph to drain away and decongest the upper respiratory tract, which subsequently helps to eliminate inflammation and reduce soreness.

Secondly, you can stimulate the healing powers of the body indirectly by massaging the neck – and we cannot overemphasise the importance of this type of massage. Running inside the upper part of the spine are two bony canals (the vertebral canals) which protect a pair of arteries known as the vertebral arteries – perhaps the most important arteries in the body after the coronary arteries in the heart. These two vertebral arteries supply blood to what is known as the inner, 'subconscious' part of the brain. Lying deep in the base of the brain, mid-brain, cerebellum and the brain stem, the subconscious brain controls your balance, gait, heartbeat, breathing, appetite, digestion, sleep, vision, hearing, smell, taste, hormones, body temperature and memory – in fact everything that is essential for your healing and wellbeing. In our opinion, poor blood flow through these vertebral arteries is responsible for many of the health problems we experience today. It is essential, therefore, regularly to reduce any stiffness in the neck, relax the muscles and decompress the upper spine – and we have developed a special massage technique to help you do this: see page 29.

the advantages of yoga

Every one of us has a healing force or sanogenetic power within us. This innate power is constantly battling inside our bodies against the factors that can make us unhealthy (such as stress, germs, excess alcohol, burning the candle at both ends) to undo any damage caused and keep us healthy. Yoga can help this process of sanogenesis. It creates a perfect feeling of wellbeing, and when the body feels good and energetic, it stimulates the body to prevent and cure illness. In fact, no other form of exercise has such a remarkable effect on the body's natural healing powers. Here are just some of the benefits of yoga:

It regulates your breathing As you'll see on pages 19–20, proper breathing is essential for a healthy life, and the art of breathing or 'pranayama' (*prana* means 'life force or energy' while *yama* means 'regulation of') is an integral part of yoga practice. By controlling your breathing, you can increase your stamina, boost your general wellbeing and improve your energy levels, alertness and clarity of mind. Breathing is therefore one of the most effective and economical ways of treating ill health.

It increases your energy Unlike more vigorous forms of exercise, which use up your reserves of energy, the slow, controlled movements of yoga – combined with effective breathing, which oxygenates the blood – actually help to generate and store energy in the body.

It stretches and works most of the muscles in the body Most physical activities are designed to tone only certain groups of muscles. Running, for example, builds up the leg and some back muscles, while weights can target specific muscles such as the biceps and triceps. So some muscles are worked to excess (which can cause repetitive strain injuries) while others are hardly used. Yoga, by contrast, takes into account all the muscles in the body, including the eye muscles, those that control swallowing, the pharyngeal muscles, the tongue, the diaphragm and many others that are rarely worked during other types of exercise. As well as being good for your general health, this can have a powerful therapeutic effect. For example, by exercising the pelvic floor muscles and anal sphincters you can help to prevent unpleasant disorders such as haemorrhoids, constipation or a prolapsed uterus.

It improves the circulation of blood and lymph The controlled muscle contractions and breathing techniques of yoga act like pumps to move blood and lymph around the body more efficiently. Certain postures improve circulation in particular parts of the body. For example, the Headstand, Shoulderstand and the Plough all increase blood and lymph flow to the heart and head. Others can direct blood towards the chest, abdomen, pelvic region, hands, feet, thyroid and so on. This increased blood flow can, in turn, improve the function of many internal organs and

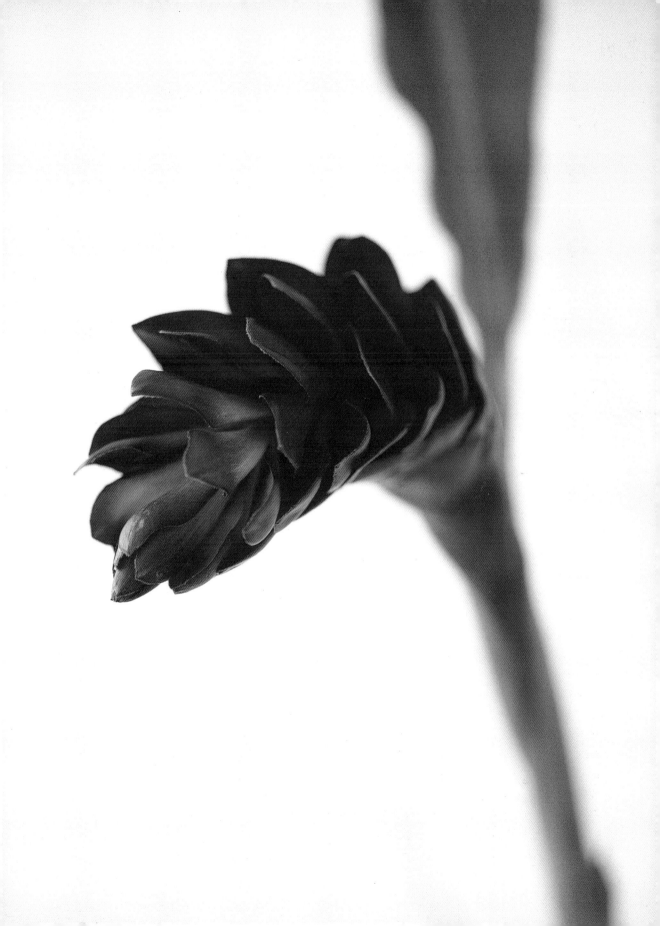

glands, such as the pancreas, ovaries, thyroid, testicles, pituitary and adrenal glands. Many diseases are caused by poor circulation, so yoga is a valuable therapeutic tool. By improving blood flow to the head, all the higher functions of the brain – including logic, concentration, memory and decision-making – are galvanised, as well as those that are responsible for the body's subconscious functions (like metabolism, reproduction, appetite and the immune response). It also helps to control the emotional centres of the brain, so yoga is very useful in managing anxiety, depression, behavioural problems and psychological illnesses.

It can exercise some involuntary muscles Through breathing and concentration, you can learn to manipulate certain muscles over which you don't normally have any control. For example, you can release the spasm of the throat muscle that causes a 'lump in the throat', prevent that knotted feeling in your stomach muscles caused by extreme nervousness or stress, reduce palpitations by controlling the heart muscles, contract the bowel muscles to improve evacuation and relax the uterine muscles during menstrual cramps.

It calms and destresses you The controlled breathing and steady movements of yoga are very good for relaxing the mind. Even experienced practitioners have to concentrate hard to synchronise their breathing with their movements, and this helps to clear the mind of all tensions. By harnessing your thoughts to a slow rhythmic pattern, you also calm the entire nervous system. After most exercises, you feel 'charged', but at the end of a session of classical yoga you feel calm and relaxed. We recommend that you always finish your yoga practice by lying in the relaxation pose known as Shavasana or the Corpse Pose, in which you control your breathing and focus your mind on different parts of your body (see pages 46–47). This position relaxes you physically after your exertions, returns your heart rate, temperature and metabolic rate to normal, brings about a state of equilibrium in the body and calms the mind. This type of post-exercise relaxation is unique to yoga.

It exercises the mind Every movement in yoga requires the participation of the conscious mind, and when complex processes such as controlled breathing, stretching, balancing, supporting the body weight and coordination are involved, different parts of the brain are switched on and off to facilitate these functions. If you do a Headstand or Shoulderstand, for example, your balance, coordination and concentration are put to extreme test as everything is upside down. All thoughts and distractions are suppressed to achieve these postures, which makes them great mental as well as physical exercise.

It improves your posture Bad posture is responsible for many common health complaints, including improper breathing, spinal problems such as backache and scoliosis, fatigue due to poor circulation and neck problems, poor muscle tone, flatulence and constipation. Yoga helps you to work on your posture – which is so essential for good health – by improving your balance and coordination and strengthening the posture-controlling muscles along the spine.

It is suitable for all ages and abilities   In fact, yoga is good for everyone! Children who practise it enjoy better health, discipline, temperament, behaviour, concentration, memory and stamina. It also facilitates their growth, prevents spinal problems such as scoliosis and improves their posture from an early age. Teenage practitioners are generally calmer and more disciplined than those who don't do yoga. They tend to outshine their peers at school and are less likely to fall into bad habits such as smoking, drinking or drug abuse. Yoga also helps to prevent many illnesses in the elderly such as backache, weak muscle tone, balance and gait disorders, constipation, fatigue, and blood pressure problems. And because it is so gentle on the heart and the body generally, it is suitable for many people advised against doing other forms of exercise, including those with heart problems, multiple sclerosis or disabilities, and those recovering from strokes or injuries.

It is safe   Most sports unfortunately entail the risk of injury, ranging from backache, sprains, stiffness and muscle strain to more serious problems such as torn cartilage, broken bones and slipped discs. The musculoskeletal system is better protected in yoga, however, as you learn to move into each posture stage by stage, over a period of time. By gradually training various groups of muscles and stretching your ligaments and joints, you can ensure you only master new postures when you – and your body – are ready.

It cleanses the body   Some of the yoga breathing exercises, particularly the cleansing breath, eliminate stagnant air in the lungs, helping to expel nicotine particles, phlegm, soot, dust and other pollutants from the lungs. Other exercises clear mucus and phlegm from the sinuses and nasal and bronchial tract, opening the passageways and reducing the risk of infections. Certain purification practices (Kriyas) are also associated with yoga, which help to cleanse various different parts of the body and flush out any toxins.

How does therapeutic yoga work?

The yoga programme recommended in the Healthy Living Routine (pages 35–47) is a general one designed to keep you in good all-round health. Therapeutic yoga goes beyond this. It focuses on individual illnesses, both chronic and acute, and cures them with tailor-made exercises. But how does it work? Well, the effects of yoga on the body can be classified into three different categories: direct, indirect, and a combination of the two. The easiest way to explain the three different effects is to look at an example of each.

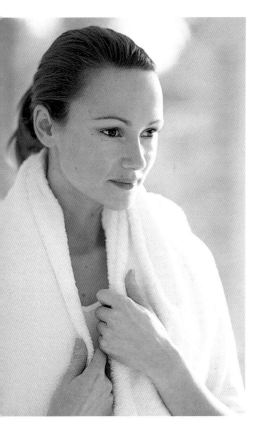

Direct effect If you have acute lower backache, you can do a series of stretching exercises to alleviate the pain and stiffness. After a few days, when your back becomes supple and more flexible, a programme of back-strengthening exercises will help to develop all the muscles whose weakness could have caused the backache in the first case. Moreover, by practising them regularly, you could prevent future attacks.

Indirect effect Take the case of a woman who has irregular periods accompanied by menstrual cramps. You might think that yoga would be of only limited help in treating this type of complaint, since irregular periods are usually the result of hormonal imbalances, and period pains tend to be caused by weakness of ligaments in the pelvic cavity that keep the uterus erect. In fact, yoga can help these sorts of conditions by working other parts of the body. Numerous yoga postures act upon the neck and improve blood flow to the base of the brain through the vertebral arteries (see page 13). These arteries supply blood to the pituitary gland, which regulates the reproductive hormones. So, by increasing blood flow to the pituitary, you improve the function of this vital gland and therefore help to normalise your menstrual cycles. In addition, many yoga postures work the lower abdomen, pelvic floor and associated internal organs; this helps to tone the muscles lining the uterus that contract to push the menstrual secretions out, reducing the pain. Moreover, yogic breathing exercises can calm the mind and reduce anxiety in the days preceding a period. This helps to ease any spasms that might occur just before menstruation is about to start. Thus yoga indirectly helps to control irregular and painful periods.

Mixed effect In the case of asthma, yoga helps directly *and* indirectly. Its direct effect is to clear the lungs and bronchial tract through breathing exercises. And indirectly it helps by improving blood flow to the pituitary gland, which mutes the body's allergic response via the adrenal glands. During an asthma attack, special breathing techniques (involving holding the breath) can also act indirectly by increasing the level of carbon dioxide in the blood; this chemical change causes the brain to release the bronchial spasm, making for slower, more comfortable breathing.

the art of breath control

Oxygen is essential to life. We can survive for a while without food or water, but not without air. We need oxygen to metabolise the food we eat and to create energy. Furthermore, breathing cools the body, supplies oxygen to all the tissues to sustain life, and expels carbon dioxide, water vapour, alcohol vapours and any other toxic gases. A lack of oxygen can cause a whole range of complaints, including headaches and dizziness, cold feet, fatigue, insomnia, food intolerances, backache, anxiety, panic attacks and muscular tension. But the good news is that you can learn to regulate your breathing, enabling the glands in your body to function more efficiently.

When you breathe in, your ribcage moves up and out (in a process known as intercostal breathing) and/or the dome of your diaphragm flattens (diaphragmatic breathing). This creates extra space in the chest cavity, producing a slight vacuum. Air then rushes into the lungs through the nostrils or the mouth. The lungs have a very rich network of capillaries, allowing the carbon dioxide in your blood to be exchanged for oxygen.

On average, people breathe 16–18 times a minute (although children may breathe slightly faster due to their higher metabolic activity). This is generally an involuntary process, meaning that most of the time you're not aware that you're doing it. Nature designed it this way because it is such a complicated process that if you had to concentrate on every movement, you would be too preoccupied to do anything else! But breathing can also be controlled to a certain extent by the conscious mind: you can hold your breath until the carbon dioxide level in your blood reaches a dangerous level and the brain takes over, forcing you to breathe again and take air into your lungs once more.

Most of us breathe too shallowly and too fast, which can unfortunately result in major health problems. This poor breathing may have a number of causes, including bad habit, stress (a major factor), and certain health problems such as dehydration, asthma and heart disease. But happily, through its stretches and breathing techniques, yoga can help to undo this damage!

Yogic breathing

When you breathe normally, only about two-thirds of the air in your lungs is expelled on exhalation and replaced when you inhale. The other third remains stagnant in your respiratory system because the lungs and the bronchial tract do not collapse totally during exhalation. When you practise yogic breathing, however, you can replace more of the air in your lungs. Yogic breathing is deeper and more efficient, and therefore more beneficial to the body.

Breath regulation is thus a crucial part of yogic practice, and is known as *pranayama*. There are a number of different *pranayama* techniques, each of which has a slightly different effect on the body. You can find details on how to perform the basic techniques on pages 32–34.

Yoga teaches you to breathe slowly and deeply, which is a great way of helping you to deal with stress. The more anxious you are, the more erratic your breathing gets. If you voluntarily slow your breathing into a deep rhythmic pattern, prolonging the time between inhalation and exhalation, oxygen absorption becomes more efficient. The blood returning to the heart from the lungs is therefore more enriched with oxygen, which triggers the brain to slow the heart rate. This can really help to calm you down. It also has other beneficial effects: it encourages the healthy functioning of your glands, which is vital for general youth and wellbeing, and by improving the oxygen supply to your brain, it helps to keep your brain cells healthy and active, which is particularly important as you grow older – your brain tissues need three times more oxygen than the rest of your body.

restorative meditation

Socrates thought that to 'know thyself' was an essential attribute of good health – and there's no better way of 'tuning in' to yourself or promoting your inner development than through meditation. The seventh limb of Patanjali's path to enlightenment (see page 8), meditation is an important part of traditional yogic practice. Contrary to popular belief, it isn't difficult to master: in fact the technique is very simple, it just takes practice. Nor is it about concentrating or controlling the mind, it just helps to increase the mind's effectiveness. It can be practised by anyone, regardless of background or faith, and certainly doesn't entail reclusiveness or a lifestyle of abstinence.

Meditation has recently been the subject of many scientific studies, and has been shown to be safe and – above all – effective in reducing anxiety, fatigue, nervousness and stress. Physiologically, it relaxes your involuntary nervous system in the same way as sleep, but you are fully awake and conscious. It is thus good at restoring both your physical and psychological health.

The idea is to focus inwards in a relaxed manner, without consciously thinking about or imagining anything in particular. At first you will probably find it quite hard to concentrate as thoughts and ideas are likely to enter your consciousness and distract you– but if you practise for about 15–20 minutes every day, you will make steady progress. There are several different schools of meditation, of which two are particularly well-known and widely practised:

Transcendental meditation This technique teaches you to repeat over and again a particular phrase or sound (a mantra), which helps to focus the mind and stop it from wandering.

Vipassana meditation Vipassana means 'to see things as they really are', and this method of meditating involves observing the breath without effort while keeping the physical body in a relaxed state.

You will benefit most from meditation through consistent, regular practice, preferably in the morning or at the same time every day. Choose a quiet environment in which to meditate, where you won't be disturbed by the phone or anything else. Sit comfortably in the lotus position or cross-legged, with your hands on top of your

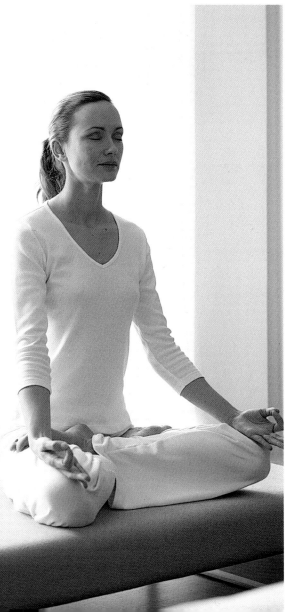

knees, palms up, and your index finger and thumb touching; this hand position increases your receptivity to knowledge and wisdom. Close your eyes, relax your body, take a few deep, slow breaths and then observe the rhythm of your breath without making an effort to breathe.

If you are practising Vipassana meditation, keep focusing on your breath and the physical sensations in your body. Choose a mantra that reflects your spiritual beliefs and continuously repeat it silently in your head. If you do find thoughts distracting you, passively observe them and then refocus on your breathing or the mantra and consciously relax your body once more. You may not be able to concentrate for very long to begin with, but with practise you will be able to meditate for longer. As a separate exercise, practise slowing down your breath; the pineal gland at the centre of your skull functions better when you have slowed your breathing down to about 4 breaths per minute. Deep meditation then occurs automatically.

At the end of your meditation, gently stroke the top of your eyelids ten times with your fingertips, working from the nose outwards. Open your eyes, remain relaxed, bow down to your inner self and carry the feeling of an open and relaxed mind throughout the day.

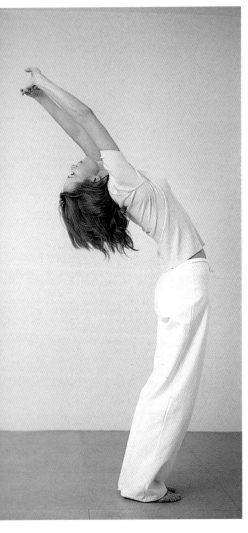

yoga in practice

If you can manage it, try to do a bit of yoga every day: aim for half an hour or more on a daily basis. The morning is the best time to practise as yoga prepares you for the day beautifully, giving you more energy, but if this isn't convenient, choose a time that suits you and try to stick to roughly the same time each day.

If you are in good health, work through the routine from Part 2 of the book; for those of you following therapeutic sequences from Part 3, alternate these with the routine. Always practise on an empty stomach (to avoid diverting blood from the digestive system where it is needed after a recent meal) and an empty bladder.

Before you begin

You don't need any expensive equipment to practise yoga: just your body and total mental presence. Wear loose, comfortable, cotton clothes that easily absorb any moisture from the body and don't restrict your movement. Remove your watch and any jewellery, and leave your feet bare.

Make sure you've got plenty of space to work in. If you have hard floors, you could consider getting a yoga mat, which helps to cushion your spine and prevents you from slipping about, or alternatively you can use a blanket or rug (provided it doesn't slide on the floor too much). Take the phone off the hook before you start and avoid distractions such as music. The room should be warm but aerated; fresh air welcomes the new day and chases away sleep and stale air.

Contraindications

If you are pregnant, suffer from very high blood pressure, chronic heart disease, retinal problems, epilepsy, or have had a joint replacement or other major surgery, you may need a yoga therapist to guide you through these exercises. It is sensible to consult your doctor, too, before beginning a yoga programme or any other form of exercise.

If you feel dizzy or light-headed during your session, especially after the breathing exercises, lie on your back and relax. This will gently improve blood flow to the brain and make you feel better. For some unknown reason, yoga can spark an uncontrolled fit of laughter or an emotional outburst in some people. If you experience this reaction after doing a few exercises, try working through the sequence of postures doing fewer repetitions, or just practise the relaxation techniques (Shavasana, or the Corpse Pose: see pages 46–47) for a couple of weeks. If the agitation persists, seek advice from a trained yoga instructor or therapist.

the principles of good practice

The most important guideline to bear in mind is always to coordinate your breathing with your movements. Breathe slowly and deeply through your nose, throughout the session. The whole idea is to regulate your breathing but not to strain it; you'll soon find that this comes naturally and that you can learn to use your breathing gently to increase a stretch safely.

The sequences of postures in Parts 2 and 3 of the book have been carefully devised to warm up, exercise and then relax your body and mind, so it is very important always to follow the order of poses as they appear. Many of the postures have been modified for people with particular ailments. Don't attempt the full pose until you are sure you can master it in proper alignment without discomfort. It is essential to listen to your body and not push it beyond its limits.

To that end, always come into and out of each position slowly and steadily. We keep emphasising the importance of regulating your breath – this is because it is easy to forget about your breathing, or even to hold your breath, which you shouldn't do when you are in a pose. So follow the step-by-step instructions carefully, as these tell you when to inhale and exhale in each position. Generally, you inhale when moving into a position and exhale to release the pose. Once you are more experienced, start holding the posture for 2–3 breaths before releasing it, as this brings about greater concentration and increases the efficiency of your body and mind to eliminate stress. To develop greater muscular strength, hold your breath for 10–12 breaths, deepening your breath as you progress. Be aware of your alignment at all times, and never force your body to stretch further than it is able.

Finally, stay relaxed! The aim is to remain mentally relaxed while stretching and strengthening your body physically. The more relaxed you are, the easier you will find it to perform the asanas, and the greater the benefits. Above all, smile while you are practising and enjoy the experience of a deeper knowledge of your body.

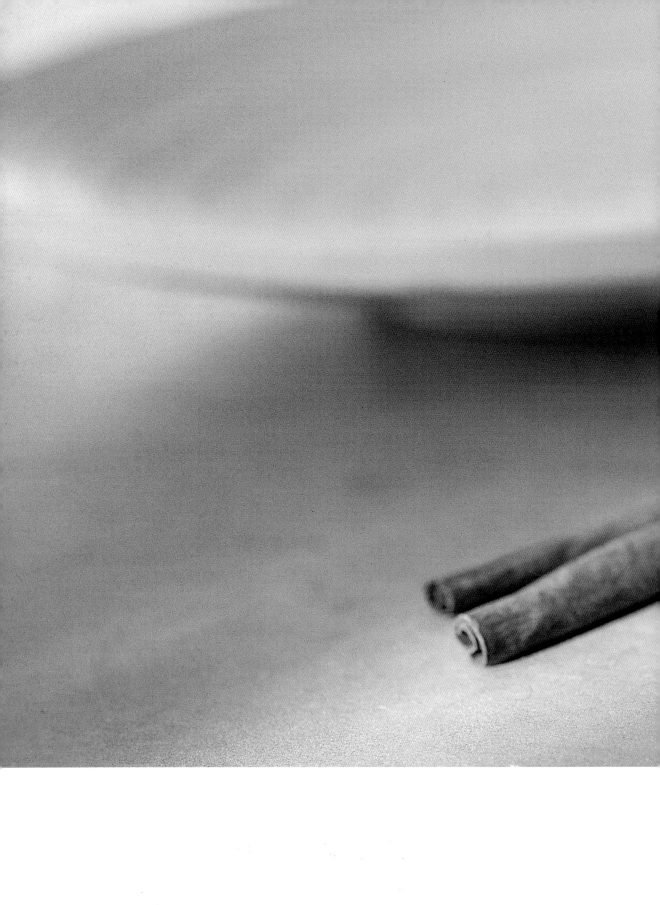

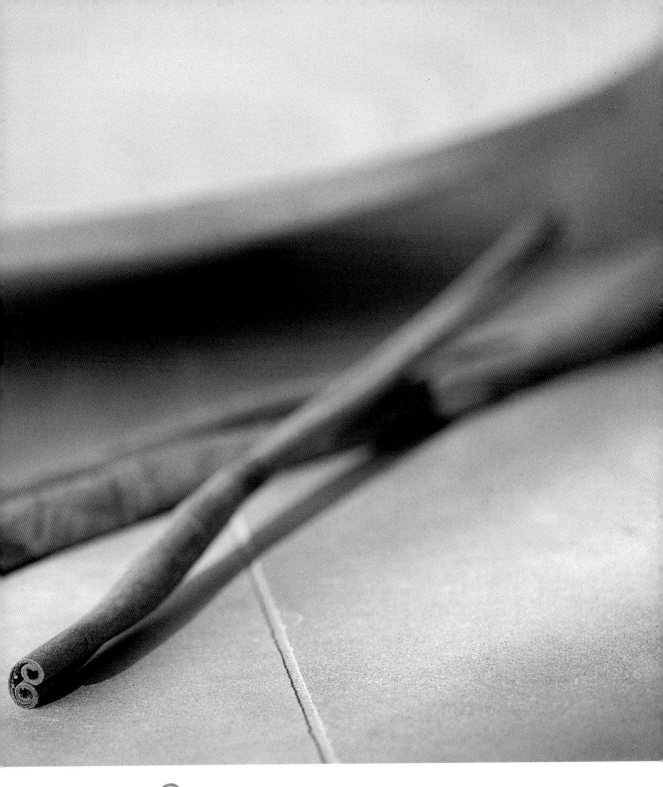

part 2 a healthy living routine

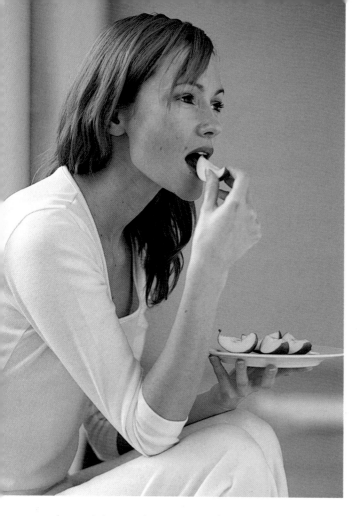

diet

Contrary to Western diet books, yogic and Ayurvedic dietary recommendations almost exclusively start with a regimen of foodstuffs and activities to avoid. Certain foods antagonise the digestive system, and for good health we recommend that you cut out or at least limit the following ingredients:

Yeast products These include bread, marmite, pizza, gravy sauces, beer, Indian nan bread, pitta bread and so on. Yeast has become a health hazard due to the overuse of antibiotics, which has led to an imbalance in the ecology that existed between bacteria, viruses and fungi. Yeast overgrowth, or candida (a mutant mould), affects digestion by excess fermentation in the gut, causing bloating. The alcohol generated by such uncontrolled fermentation is often toxic, producing fatigue, skin rash, diarrhoea and other symptoms.

Sour or stomach-acid-producing substances Limit your intake of citrus fruits, wine, spirits, very spicy food, nuts, excessive painkillers or anti-inflammatory drugs, tobacco, canned products containing citric acid as a preservative and deep-fried food (the oil coats the stomach lining causing the amount of acid in the stomach to increase). Excess stomach acid interferes with the digestion in the duodenum, where the finer digestion takes place, by neutralising the total bile content secreted into the duodenum. As a result the food pulp in the duodenum remains stagnant or undigested until more bile is secreted. When this happens you can feel heavy and bloated. Excess stomach acid also causes heartburn when it regurgitates or spills out, and can cause gastritis (inflammation of the stomach lining) and even ulcers.

Excess alcohol No matter how much money wine-growers may put into research that suggests that wine is good for the heart, mind and body, too much alcohol is bad for you. Firstly, there is the question of addiction. Secondly, alcohol gets metabolised mainly in the liver, where it deprives the precious liver cells of oxygen. These liver cells therefore malfunction, and ultimately scar tissue grows into the liver tissue causing cirrhosis, an irreversible condition. The liver processes all of the digested food entering from the gut and manufactures numerous chemicals and enzymes for the body. Liver damage would slowly poison the body and fail to supply it with essential ingredients.

Excess coffee Caffeine overstimulates the nervous system. The body becomes tense and your heart rate and breathing rate go up, as if you were ready for a 'fight or flight' stress reaction. Coffee is therefore incompatible with yoga, which tries to calm the body down.

Cheese and mushrooms Cheese causes excess mucus production in the nasal and bronchial tract. It also contains moulds that, like mushrooms, produce gas. Mushrooms and moulds contain toxins that are potentially bad for the body. Some mushrooms can kill, and we all know that penicillin, the mother of all antibiotics, is a mould product. Fungi are parasites and therefore deprive the body of essential nutrients, as they compete for finer foods.

Canned and preserved foods Canned foods contain preservatives to stop bacterial and fungal growth. Some preservatives, such as sugar (common as a syrup in tinned fruits) and vinegar (present in some sauces and juices) are less harmful than the chemical ones. Don't be misled by an 'organic' label on canned products and think that the foods are free of preservatives. An 'organic' label guarantees its source, certifying that the foods were organically grown, but this doesn't mean that there are no chemicals or preservatives in them, however small the quantities may be.

Fizzy water This interferes with peristalsis, or movement of the intestines, as the gas stretches their walls like a balloon.

Chocolates, sweets and desserts In excess, sugary foods slow down the digestive process by 'feeding' the gut yeast, causing fermentation. Some of the alcohols produced by gut fermentation are toxic, and can cause lethargy, skin irritation, abdominal discomfort and other unpleasant effects.

Fried and oily foods These take a long time to digest and therefore put an extra burden on the digestive system. Besides that, they add to the weight problem.

Rich curries and very spicy food Spicy foods (especially with excess chillies) are very addictive. The hot taste dilates your blood vessels, flushes the face and the head, makes the mouth water, creates appetite (by increasing the secretion of digestive juices) and increases the heart rate. All these act as a 'kick' – but hot food causes excess salivation and stomach acid (heartburn).

massage

Ideally, try to have a massage at least once a week – you can either perform it yourself or get someone else (a friend, partner or a professional masseur) to do it for you. The only equipment you need is a couple of towels for cushioning and to cover any areas of the body not being massaged, and some massage oil. The best time for a massage is 2–3 hours after a meal. Make sure the room is nice and warm, then put on some soft music and you are ready to begin.

Massage strokes

Before making contact with the skin, remove your watch and any jewellery that might get in the way. Make sure your fingernails won't snag, too. Always pour a little massage oil into your palms first and warm it up by rubbing your hands together. The following massage routines use two main types of contact: friction and pressure.

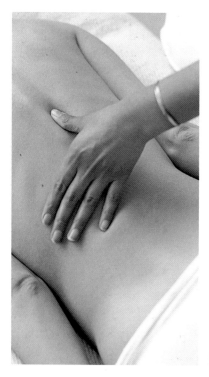 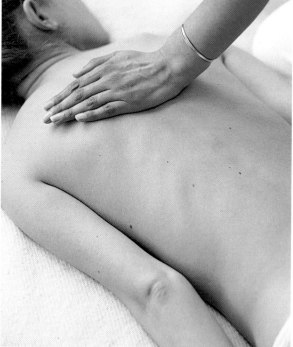

Pressure Use your thumbs or fingertips to work deep into the tissue and feel for any knotted or sore spots.

Friction Rub the palms of your hands across the surface of the skin – either in straight lines or circular movements – to invigorate the muscles and encourage blood flow.

Self-massage

This can be a great way to relieve aches and pains as and when they occur, and the neck massage in particular is very effective at improving blood flow to the brain. The best time to massage yourself is an hour before a bath, perhaps at the weekend when you're properly relaxed. Set aside about 15 minutes for the massage. Alternatively, you can do it while you're actually in the bath, using massage oil or even shower gel as a lubricant, and focus just on your neck and shoulders.

Put a towel on the floor and sit on it with your legs wide in front of you. The best oils to use are Dr Ali's Lifestyle Oil (100 ml apricot or grapeseed oil; 30 drops lavender; 30 drops geranium; 30 drops ylang ylang) or compressed sesame oil; rub a teaspoon or so in your palms and you are ready to begin. You'll need about 4 tablespoons of oil altogether: at the end of the massage your skin should have acquired a soft texture without being greasy. Have a bath or shower an hour or two later.

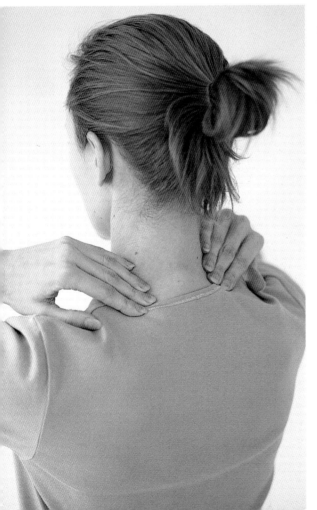

1 Start by massaging the muscles in your neck, shoulders and as much as you can reach of your upper back. You'll find several areas of tenderness in the neck. Massage these deeply using your thumbs or fingers.

2 Squeeze the shoulder area for 2–3 seconds and then release. If there are any knots or sore spots, try to disperse them by massaging more deeply.

3 Then concentrate on your jaws for 1–2 minutes.

4 Move on to your shoulder joints and then rub your biceps and down to your wrists.

5 Use your thumbs to massage your palms and then entwine your fingers together and massage the areas between your fingers.

6 Then reach behind and massage what you can of your lower back, particularly your buttocks, and move down to your thighs, calves and feet. Concentrate on your calves as a lot of tension (in the form of lactic acid) accumulates here. Squeeze your calves and massage down towards your Achilles tendons and the ankles.

7 Finally, use your thumbs to massage the soles of your feet and your toes.

Partner massage

Certain parts of the body, such as the back and neck, are more easily reached by someone else, so team up with a friend or partner and take turns to treat each other to a massage. The best time to give or receive a massage is at bedtime as it induces sleep by reducing muscle fatigue and improving blood flow to the brain. Have your partner lie on his or her front with a pillow or cushion under the chest so that the head and neck are suspended over it.

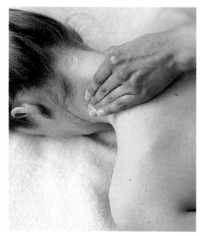

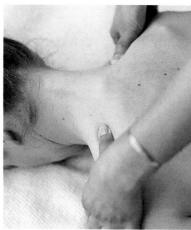

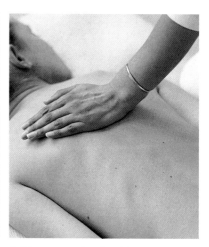

1 Massage the neck and shoulder area thoroughly. Using your thumb on one side of the neck and your fingers on the other, massage all the muscles and tendons up and down. Then squeeze the muscles and draw your thumbs and fingers closer to the centre.

2 Work on the entire length of the muscles from the skull to the shoulder region. There will be a few areas of tenderness, particularly on one side. Massage these areas deeply, even if it hurts a little, releasing the tension.

3 Move on to the shoulders, pressing the trapezius muscles on top of and between the shoulder blades to relieve all the spasms. Concentrate on this area for about 5 minutes.

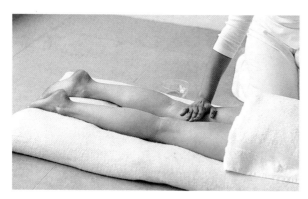

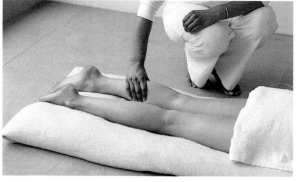

7 Still using the balls of your hands, massage the hamstrings at the back of the thighs. Start at the seat area, and slide your hands down towards the ankles, increasing the pressure with each stroke. You'll feel the tense muscles relaxing.

8 Work down the calves and all the way to the ankles. Squeeze and release the muscles in the calves until they feel thoroughly relaxed. Finish by massaging the soles of the feet with your thumbs.

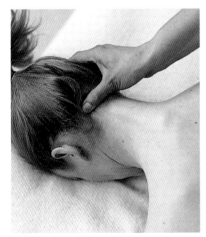

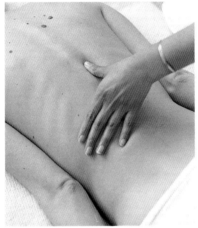

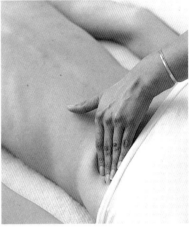

4 Now work on the jaws and temples, where a lot of tension is retained. Massage the back of the base of the skull where the tendons of the neck muscles are attached. These are often quite tender.

5 Use one or both thumbs to massage the long muscles of the back, which are located about 3–4 cm away from the centre of the spine. Start at the bottom of the spine and push right up to the top, repeating for 2 or 3 minutes.

6 With the help of your thumbs or fingers, massage along the sides of the back, working from the centre of the spine outwards. From here move on to the gluteal or buttock region and press deeply for a couple of minutes in a circular motion.

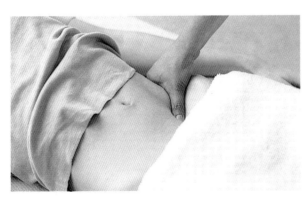

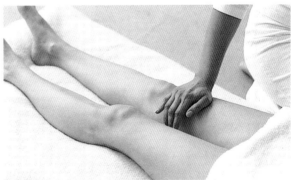

9 Ask the person receiving the massage to turn over. Then, using your thumb or fingers, work into the fleshy area on top of the pelvic bone for a couple of minutes.

10 To finish, press on the top of the thighs with the ball of your hand and slide down to the knee, increasing the pressure with each stroke. Any tension in the thigh muscles will start to dissipate.

breath control

The art of yogic breathing, known as pranayama, is an integral part of yoga practice, and the key to improving your physiological and psychological wellbeing (see pages 19–20). Using the diaphragm (the main breathing muscle in the body) independently of movements in the spine is an essential skill to develop.

There are a number of different breathing techniques, but most consist of the same three basic components:

Inhalation This should be smooth and continuous and prolonged over time to assist in expanding your lung capacity.

Retention of (or holding) the breath after inhalation This has a cleansing effect on the body as it allows time for fresh air to mix with the stale air in your lungs, and also permits a greater absorption of oxygen into the blood. You should therefore aim to prolong this retention for as long as is possible.

Exhalation This is a passive process in which the lungs recoil and the chest relaxes. It should be continuous, relaxed and complete. A natural suspension of breath can sometimes occur after complete exhalation, which produces a state of deep tranquillity.

The whole idea is to strengthen your breathing so that you require fewer breaths per minute. Aim initially for a ratio of 1:1:1 of inhaling, holding and exhaling. Gradually increase this to 1:1:2. Advanced practice allows for a ratio of 1:4:2, but this is only for experienced practitioners. Once you can slow your breathing to about 8 breaths per minute, your pituitary gland (the master gland in your brain which controls the secretions of all the other glands in your body) will be at its most efficient. But if, at any point when you are working through the breathing exercises that involve holding your breath, you feel flushed or your heart rate goes up, breathe naturally until you are ready to try holding your breath again.

Some breathing methods are recommended for daily use (see the yoga programme on pages 35–47), others have wonderful therapeutic effects and are therefore recommended later in the book under specific ailments. Whichever breathing technique you are using, however, don't forget always to breathe through your nose. This has many advantages: the tiny hairs in the nasal passage act as a natural filter for dust particles, pollen, germs and other nasties, and help to keep the nasal tract moist. What's more, nasal breathing warms up cold air before it enters the lungs and minimises the likelihood of developing sinus congestion. By contrast, breathing through the mouth can cause dryness in the mouth and a congested feeling in the forehead. If your nose is blocked, try to clear it with a nasal douche (see page 73).

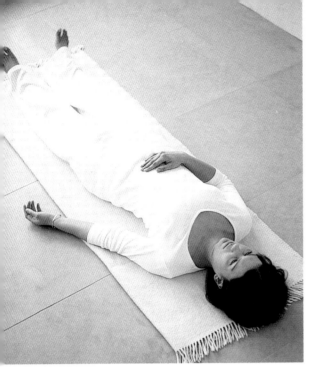

Abdominal Breathing
Pranayama

By moving the diaphragm, this exercise gently massages your internal organs and relaxes the lower abdominal area, thereby improving the blood flow through all the muscles and nerve centres.

1 Lie on your back and relax your arms, legs, head and neck completely. Breathe in through your nose and extend your stomach completely, like a balloon filled with air. Avoid arching your back.

2 Breathe out slowly and let your stomach relax. Do not try to pull your stomach muscles in at this stage. Repeat for at least 20 breaths.

Complete Breath
Ujjayi Pranayama

This technique helps to increase your lung capacity, to relieve tension in your upper spine and to open out the mid-chest, decongesting the area.

1 Stand or sit cross-legged on the floor. First, breathe out completely. When you inhale, relax your diaphragm by letting go of the area below the ribcage and fill up your lungs slowly and steadily by expanding your chest up and out. Visualise every part of your lungs filling up with air.

2 Now exhale slowly. Try to make your out-breath longer than your in-breath, but stay comfortable. Don't pull in your abdomen – let it relax by itself, so that your lungs remain passive as they empty. Continue for 10 minutes, maintaining the same position and rhythm of breath throughout.

3 When you can perform Steps 1 and 2 without strain, try to hold your breath to achieve a ratio between inhalation, holding and exhalation of 1:1:2. Repeat 20 such breaths. Lie down and relax in the Corpse Pose (see pages 46–47).

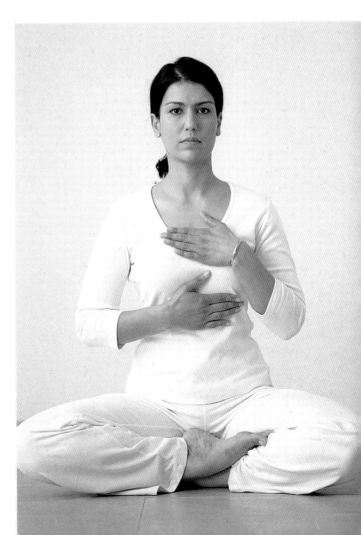

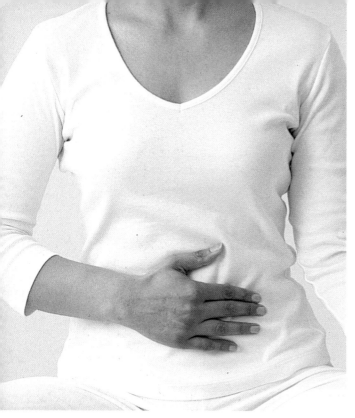

Alternate Nostril Breathing

Anuloma-Viloma Pranayama

This exercise helps you to control the heating and cooling mechanisms in your body. Breathing through the right nostril creates heat, vitality and alertness, while breathing through the left one has a cooling effect. The pituitary gland in the brain controls this natural thermostat within your body, although its functioning can be disrupted through an insufficient blood supply. This breathing technique allows you to regulate your thermostat more consciously.

1 Sit cross-legged if possible or on a straight-backed chair. Tuck the index and middle fingers of your right hand into your palm as shown below or simply use your thumb and index finger. Place your thumb on your right nostril to close it and breathe in deeply through your left nostril.

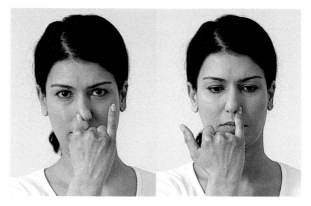

Cleansing Breath

Kapalabhati

As well as being a pranayama, Kapalabhati is one of the six Kriyas or purification methods. Here, exhalation is brief and active – the abdominals are contracted sharply to expel stale air. This dislodges excess mucus from the lungs, increases oxygen uptake in the body and strengthens nerve cells. Omit this exercise if you have high blood pressure, a hernia, an ulcer, prolapsed organs in the lower abdomen, or suffer from eye or ear complaints.

1 Stand or sit comfortably with your arms relaxed by your sides. Straighten your upper back and pull your shoulders back. Close your mouth and look straight ahead. Breathe in fully through your nose.

2 Breathe out quickly, pulling your stomach in. Pause between breaths for a second or so, and then breathe in again, taking your time. Repeat 25 times.

3 Lie down and relax in the Corpse Pose (see pages 46–47) for at least 10 minutes.

2 Close your left nostril with your finger and release your thumb. Breathe out completely through your right nostril. Feel your chest muscles relaxing and your shoulders dropping away from your neck as you exhale. Then breathe in through your right nostril.

3 Close your right nostril, release your finger and breathe out through the left one. You have now completed 1 cycle. Continue for 3–5 minutes.

4 Lie down on your back and relax in the Corpse Pose (see pages 46–47).

yoga programme

The sequence of yoga exercises described on the following pages has been specially devised to promote your general wellbeing and enhance your willpower. This increases your energy levels and disciplines your mind so you will enjoy better health and stay looking younger!

If you can, try to work through the sequence on a daily basis. You will gain the greatest benefits from these poses if you bear the following points in mind:

Always coordinate your movements with your breath   You can use Ujjayi breathing or relaxed Abdominal Breathing (see page 33) throughout your yoga practice. Aim to slow down your breathing in each posture as you improve. Listen to your body and relax if you feel the overwhelming need to do so between postures.

You shouldn't feel any strain   If your breathing is no longer rhythmical, it is a sign of stress, so go back a stage in the physical posture and regulate your breath. This is a sure way to prevent injury and gain deeper relaxation.

Take it easy   Always release a big stretch slowly, again keeping your breathing slow and steady. Pull your spine upwards in all positions, creating a lightness in your body. As your muscles strengthen, aim to stay in each posture for 12 breaths. Relax your jaw area throughout by dropping your tongue from the roof of your mouth.

Watch your alignment   In standing positions, ensure that your feet point straight ahead, in line with your ankles (rather than turning them out); your ankles should be below your knees, your knees below your hips, your hips below your shoulders and your shoulders should be in line with your ears. Gently pull your shoulders back without overarching your spine, and keep your neck straight; don't jut your chin out or up – it should be in line with your eyes. Your palms should be by the sides of your thighs. When squatting down, remember always to bend your knees over your toes. When stretching the spine in sitting positions, your knees should face upwards and not outwards. And if you are reaching forwards, bend from your hips and not your upper back. As you begin to stretch the main joints, all these aspects of alignment will become easier to watch.

Be wary of overstretching   This can misalign your body and you may have to increase the strength of your postural muscles much more to maintain good posture. Remember, the stretching you do here releases tension in your joints and strengthens your muscles. This balances the contraction and relaxation levels of the muscles on either side of a joint creating greater stability wthin the body.

Enjoy yourself   Be sure to remember that yoga is all about achieving a relaxed state of mind and an enhanced perception of your body and mind.

The Locomotive
Hrd Gati

This exercise warms you up and is good for those with hyperextended knees. If you find it too complicated, march on the spot instead, moving your arms backwards and forwards and lifting your knees as high as you comfortably can.

1   Stand up straight with your feet slightly apart and bend your arms at the elbows. Step forward onto your left leg, aiming to hit your buttocks with your right heel, and move your right arm forward.

2   Now step onto your right foot and reverse the arm position. Keep moving forwards for about 50 steps, pushing your arms backwards and forwards like the pistons on a steam train. Breathe in and out deeply throughout.

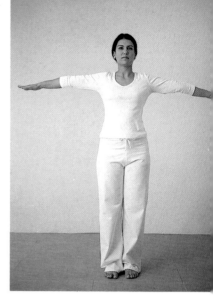

Back Strengthener I
Kati Sakti Vikasaka

1   Stand up straight with your feet slightly apart and lift your arms out to the sides at shoulder level with your palms facing down. Keep your arms taut.

2   Breathe in, and bend to the right from your waist. Breathe out and come back up. Now breathe in and bend over to the left. Repeat 10 times on each side without moving your arms.

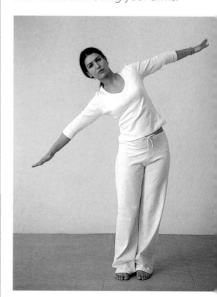

Back Strengthener II
Kati Sakti Vikasaka

1 Stand up straight and place your hands on the top of your buttocks. Press your shoulders back. Take a deep breath in and arch backwards, taking care not to throw your neck back, and look up comfortably.

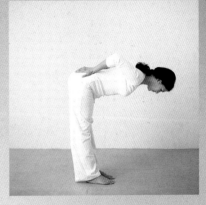

2 Exhale and stretch forwards comfortably. Aim over time to create a 90° angle between your torso and legs. Keep your back and neck straight. Repeat 5 times slowly.

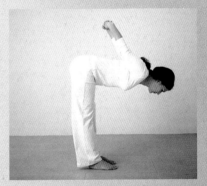

3 Repeat Step 2, but this time interlock your hands behind you and stretch your arms up on bending forward. Be very gentle as this is a more intense variation. To finish, come up on your toes, and then squat down with your hands on the floor for a few breaths.

Spinal Rock
Pindasana

1 Lie on your back, making sure your shoulders and hips are relaxed towards the floor. Bend your legs, bring your knees up to your chest and cross your ankles. Now cross your wrists in front of your body and start to reach for your ankles; your arms should be in-between your knees.

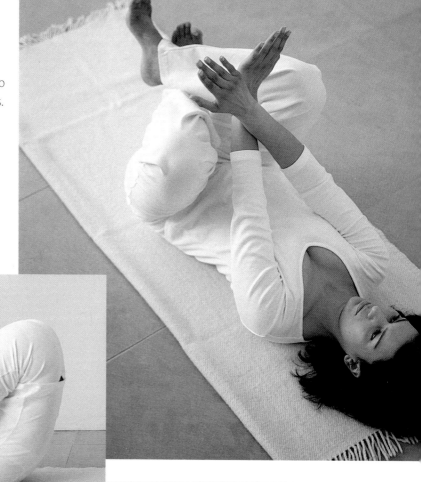

2 Holding onto your ankles, gently rock backwards and forwards on your rounded back. Breathe out as you roll backwards onto your upper spine, and breathe in as you roll forwards until your feet touch the floor. Repeat about 10 times.

3 When you've mastered Step 2, sit up on going forwards, cross your legs and gently stretch forwards. Then roll back again, taking care not to let go of your ankles.

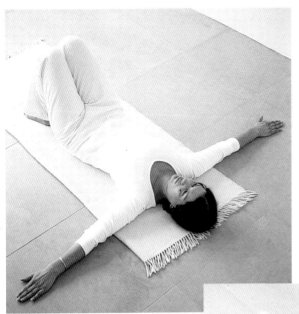

Supine Twist I
Supta Parivritasana

1. Lie down on your back with your arms out to the sides at shoulder level and your feet together on the floor, your knees bent.

2. Breathe in, then breathe out and pull in your stomach strongly towards your spine. Lift your knees up to your chest and then lower them towards the floor on the right, at a right angle to your torso. Hold the position and breathe rhythmically, relaxing your upper body completely. Stay for 2–3 breaths, working up to 12 breaths. Then bring your knees up to your chest once more and lower them to the left.

3. As you become more flexible, repeat Step 2 with your hands under your head. Finish by bringing your knees to your chest – this is called the Embryo Pose. Having freed up the chest and main joints, stand up or sit in Siddhasana (cross-legged) to do a few short Kapalabhati breaths (see page 34).

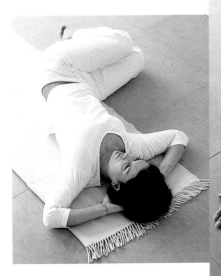

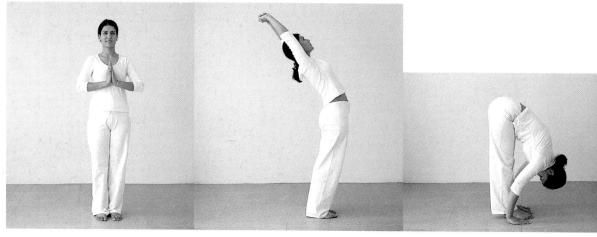

1 Stand with your feet together (or hip-width apart if you find it easier) and your palms together in front of your chest. Distribute your weight evenly. Take a few slow, deep breaths and keep your shoulders down and your neck straight. Avoid arching your mid-spine; tuck your abdomen in towards the spine.

2 Take a deep breath in, relax the area below the ribcage and expand your ribs outwards and forwards. Lift up your arms and stretch back, pushing your hips forwards but keeping your legs straight. Look up. If you have a weak, painful neck, look straight ahead and just stretch up your arms.

3 Breathe out slowly and fold forwards, pulling your arms in front of you before reaching down to place your palms on the floor. Your hands should remain in this position for the rest of the sequence. Lower your head towards your shins, relaxing your neck. If you can, straighten your legs; if your back is stiff, bend your knees a little. If your wrists are painful, place your knuckles on the floor.

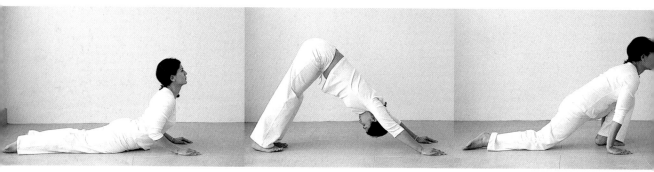

7 Breathe in and lower your hips to the floor. Point your toes and then stretch back. Press your shoulders down (you may need to bend your elbows), keep your upper back straight, push your chest forwards and look up.

8 Breathe out, curl your toes under again and lift your hips to form an upside-down 'V'. Stretch your heels down gently to touch the floor and relax your head down. Stretch out your arms and keep your spine straight.

9 Breathe in and step your left foot forwards in-between your hands. Rest your right knee on the ground and straighten your neck, as in Step 4.

Salute to the Sun **Surya Namaskar**

You should ideally perform this graceful cycle of 12 basic postures in the morning, to prepare you for the day ahead. Work through the series slowly, coordinating your breathing with each movement. Use Ujjayi breathing (see page 33) throughout. The aim is to reduce the number of breaths required to complete the cycle. For an aerobic workout, repeat for 20 minutes.

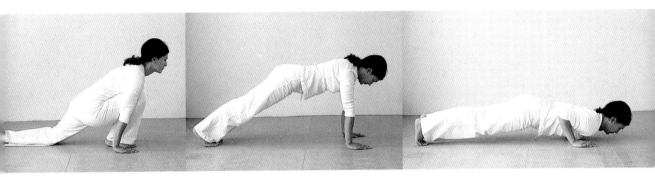

4 | Breathe in and take your left leg back, resting the knee on the floor, with your toes curled under. Stretch your right knee forward while keeping the heel on the floor. Straighten your upper back and neck.

5 | Hold your breath and take your right foot back to join the left one. Support your weight on your hands and toes. Keep your spine in line with your head and look at the space in-between your hands.

6 | Breathe out and lower your knees towards the floor by bending your arms. If your arms can't hold you, lower your knees to the floor first. Now lower your chest and forehead to the ground without dropping your hips.

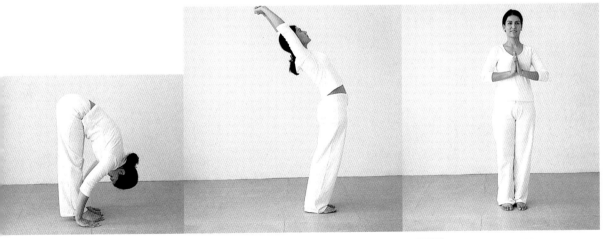

10 | Breathe out, bring your right foot forwards besides the left one, straighten your legs and fold forwards, as in Step 3. Try to bend from the hips and not the upper back.

11 | Breathe in, stretch your arms out in front of you and then lift up and stretch back, as in Step 2.

12 | Breathe out and lower your arms into the prayer position as shown. Stand straight and tall, distributing your weight evenly. You've completed 1 round. Repeat 2 rounds initially, building gradually to 12 rounds.

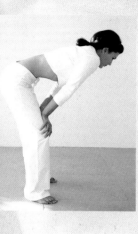

Abdominal Lock

Uddiyana Bandha

This is a must for any yogic practice. It stimulates digestion, encourages peristaltic action of the intestines and massages the liver and spleen as well as contributing to the strength of the abdominals.

1 Stand with your feet hip-width apart. Bend forward with your hands on your knees. Take a deep breath in. Breathe out through your mouth, emptying your lungs.

2 Without inhaling, pull in your stomach and then lift it up towards the ribcage. Hold for a count of 5, increasing this to 10 seconds over time. Let go and relax your breath. Repeat 5 times. Gradually, try to pump your stomach in and out 5 times without breathing in.

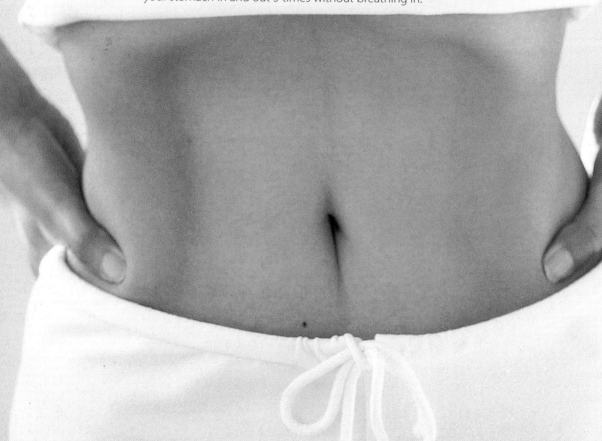

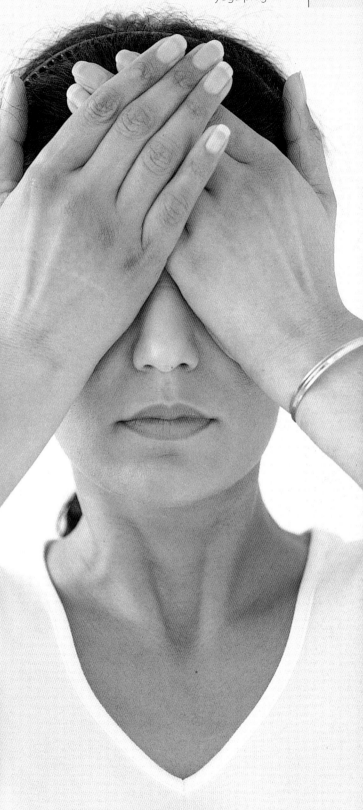

Palming

Netra Sakti Vikasaka

This is a great exercise for relaxing the eyes. The longer you do it, the greater the benefits. Seeing perfect black on palming indicates perfect relaxation. If you can't see black, you will only increase the strain. Try improving your eyes with some of the other eye exercises and then come back to palming.

1 Sit comfortably with your shoulders relaxed and your neck straight; relax your breathing. Rotate your eyes in a clockwise direction 5 times and then anti-clockwise 5 times. This gently stimulates the muscles controlling eye movement.

2 Close your eyes. Rub your palms together vigorously to create warmth and place them over your closed eyes for at least a count of 10, with your fingers crossing your forehead to ensure proper palming. Relax your facial muscles. Repeat if necessary.

3 Look straight ahead, keeping your eyes relaxed. Then look up for a count of 5 before looking straight ahead and relaxing the eyes. Look down for a count of 5, then look straight ahead and relax the eyes. Look up diagonally to the right, down to the left, and then straight ahead and relax the eyes. Look up diagonally to the left, down to the right, and then straight ahead and relax the eyes. Lastly, close your eyes and repeat the palming in Step 2 to relax your eyes and mind.

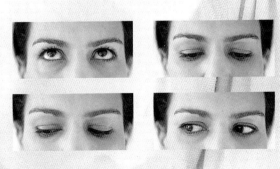

Central Fixation

Tratak

Tratak is a Kriya (one of the six purification methods) and involves gently gazing at a point without blinking, and then closing the eyes to visualise the point. As well as helping to treat glaucoma, incipient cataract and inflammation of the iris, Tratak also improves concentration, stills the mind and boosts the memory. It helps to relax the facial muscles too, smoothing away wrinkles and dark circles around the eyes.

1 Light a candle and place it about 1.5 m away from you at eye level. Sit in a relaxed position, take a few deep, slow breaths, then relax the breath to a steady rhythm. With your eyes open but relaxed, gaze at the flame without blinking. If you do blink, relax and start again. You should aim to gaze at the flame without blinking until tears begin to flow. Then close your eyes and visualise the shape of the flame on your forehead.

2 You can also perform Tratak by gazing at the middle of your forehead or at the tip of your nose.

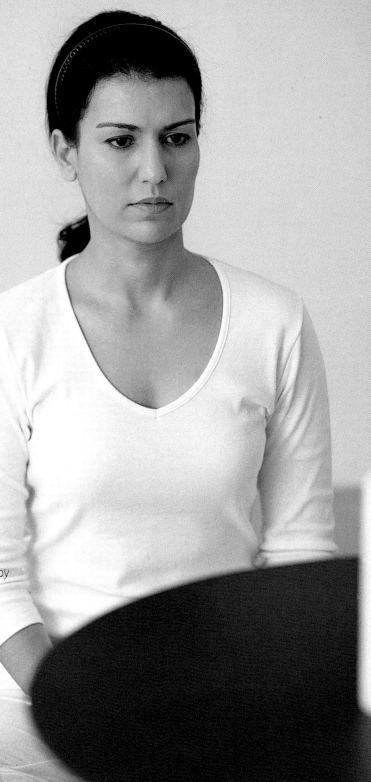

Swinging
Kati Chakrasana

This will help to improve your vision and relieve fatigue. With continual practice, you should be able to swing without effort, and a feeling of relaxation will take over in the muscles and nerves of the body.

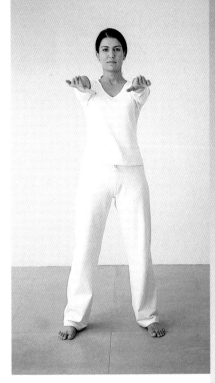

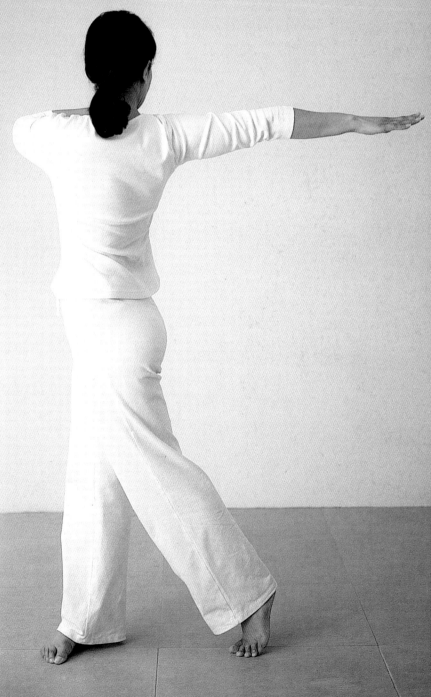

1   Stand with your feet about 30 cm apart. Raise your arms up in front of you at shoulder level.

2   Swing to the right by lifting your left heel a little off the floor until your shoulders are in line behind you. Keep your right arm straight while you bend your left arm. Now reverse and swing to the left. Continue swinging from one side to the other, paying attention to moving your head and eyes with your shoulders. As you swing, try not to focus your eyes on any of the objects that appear to be moving rapidly in front of you. Repeat 50 times before going to bed and on waking up in the morning.

Neck Rolls

Griva Sakti Vikasaka

Neck exercises are always useful at night-time for a refreshing sleep.

1 Sit comfortably on a chair, on your heels or cross-legged on the floor. Lower your chin and slowly rotate your neck, first to the right and then to the left, breathing deeply.

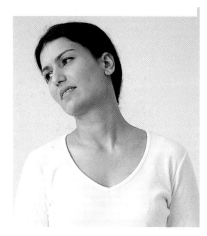

2 Finish by inhaling and lowering your chin to your sternum; hold your breath for at least 10 seconds. This is known as Jalandhara Bandha. Release slowly on exhaling, relaxing the shoulders.

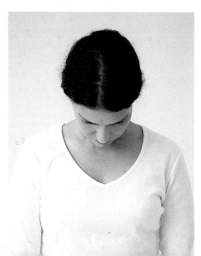

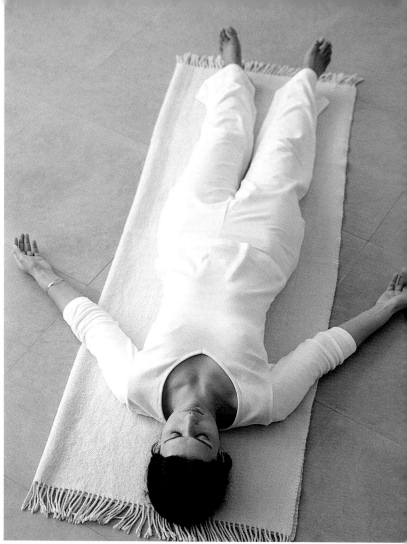

Corpse Pose

Shavasana

This may sound easy, but it is in fact the most difficult posture to achieve because it's hard to let your muscles relax as if you were in a deep sleep while remaining conscious. Steps 2–4 gently stretch the back and sides of the neck and the shoulders, which helps to relax the whole body.

1 Lie on your back with your feet apart and your legs relaxing outwards; keep your arms a little away from your trunk, palms up. Take a deep breath in and stretch the back of your neck away from your shoulders by lowering your chin. Breathe out slowly and let go of the neck and shoulders, allowing them to 'sink' towards the floor. Relax your facial muscles. Your abdomen should rise on inhaling and fall on exhaling.

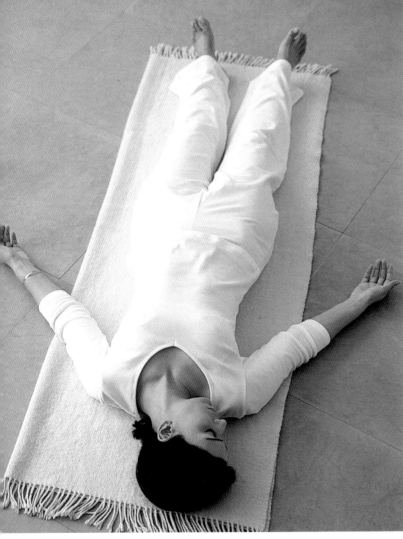

5. Now, just lie still and let your mind's eye wander over your body, starting with the toes. Keep your breathing below the ribcage: it should be rhythmic, smooth and light without any constrictions. Relax your muscles completely. Try to let the base of the skull sink deeper and deeper towards the floor. Then check your breathing again. Stay in this posture for 20 minutes.

6 Slowly turn to the right with your right hand under your head. Relax, then slowly roll over and repeat on the left. Turn to the right again to stand up slowly.

2 Take another deep breath in, lift your arms up and stretch them out on the ground behind your head. Flex your toes to stretch the back of the legs. Breathe out slowly and relax your arms, feet, legs and neck. Go back to normal breathing. Slowly lower your arms to your sides again.

3 Take a deep breath in and press your shoulders down away from your neck. Stretch your fingers out and point to your toes with your out-stretched arms. Breathe out slowly and relax again. Go back to observing normal breath.

4 Now breathe in and turn your head to the right so that your right ear is touching the floor. Keep your left shoulder pressed down to the floor. Maintain this stretch on breathing out. Now go back to normal breathing. Relax the left side of your neck and shoulders. Stay in this position for 2–3 minutes, relaxing your facial muscles, particularly the jaw, by taking your tongue away from the roof of your mouth. Repeat on the other side.

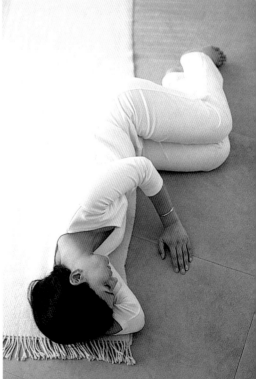

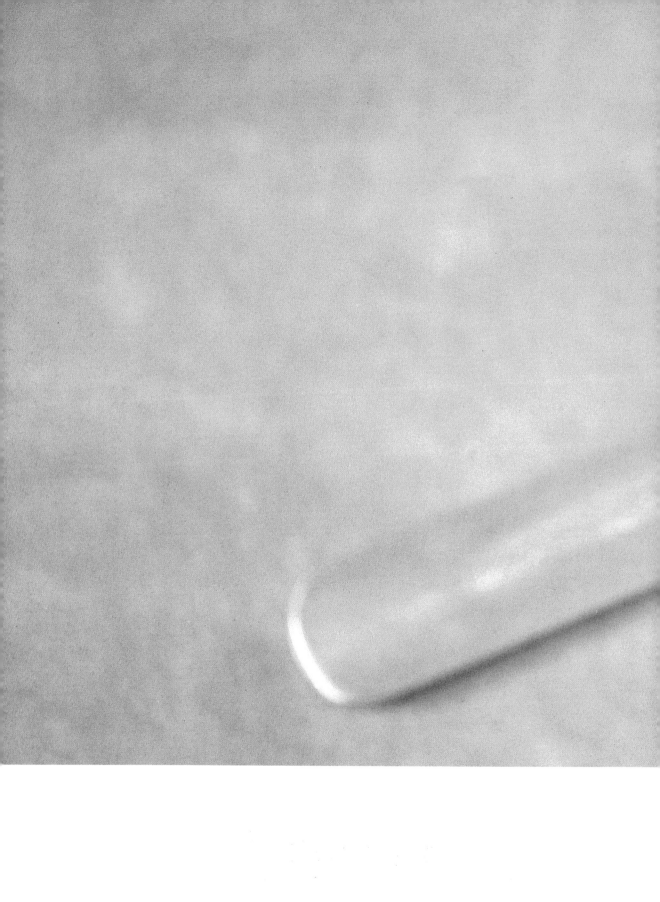

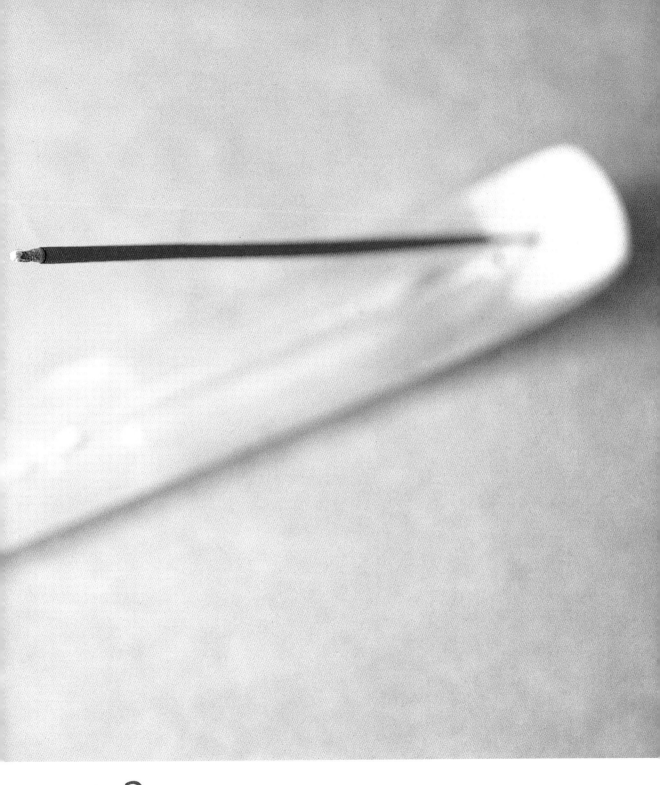

part 3 yoga therapy

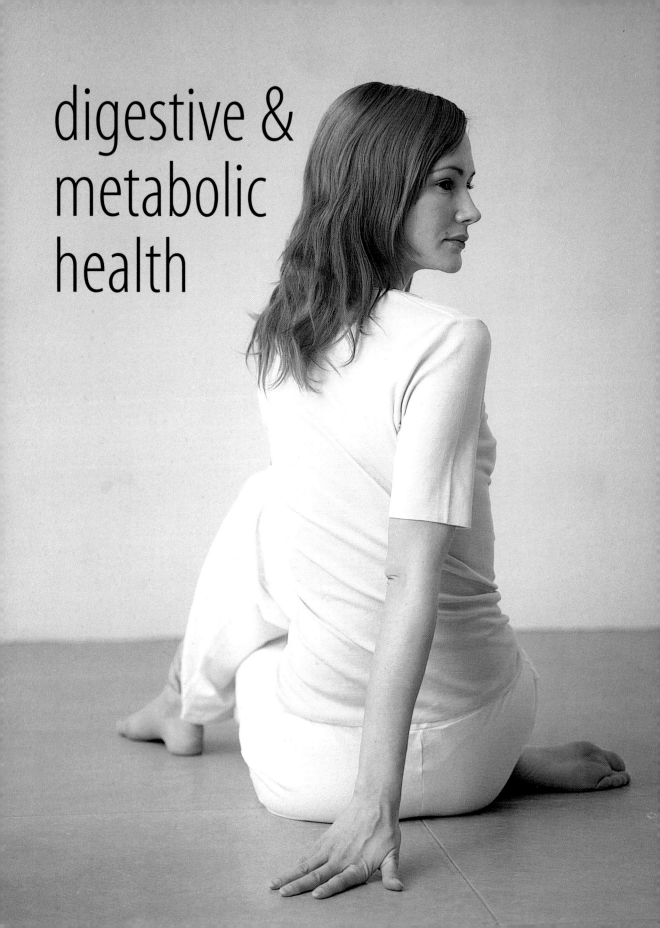

digestive & metabolic health

irritable bowel syndrome

This is a common abdominal condition characterised by a group of symptoms, including abdominal pain or cramps, constipation and/or diarrhoea, flatulence, bloating, acidity (heartburn), nausea and vomiting. The precise cause of irritable bowel syndrome (IBS) is unknown, although certain foods, *Candida* and stress may be triggers.

Because the mechanism of irritable bowel syndrome is poorly understood, the effectiveness of conventional medical treatment (often involving the prescription of antidepressants) is limited. By contrast, many complementary physicians have excelled in treating IBS because they take a more holistic approach. According to complementary wisdom, IBS may be caused by an overgrowth of *Candida albicans* (a yeast-like fungus) in the digestive system. The fungus exists naturally on the surface of certain areas of the body such as the mouth and throat, but sometimes it can grow out of control or spread to other areas of body, where it causes problems. If *Candida* develops in the digestive system, it can make microscopic holes in the wall of the gut, which allow undesirable molecules to enter the gut and destroy the immunological balance of the digestive system. Complementary therapists therefore regulate the diet very cautiously to aid digestion and bring relief from many symptoms of IBS. They also introduced the system of replacing the gut flora with beneficial bacteria such as *Lactobacillus acidophyllus* and *Lactobacillus bifidus*, which inhibit the growth of harmful bacteria.

Our approach to IBS is very general, designed to improve your digestion overall and not just treat individual symptoms. One of the ways we do this is by realigning the solar plexus. This is a network of nerve fibres located in the centre of the abdomen, from which radiate nerves to the gall bladder, stomach and intestines. Because it controls so many of the digestive organs, it can cause all sorts of abdominal problems if it gets entangled, twisted or moved. The position of the solar plexus can be determined by the position of the navel or belly button, and experienced therapists can realign it through a special manipulation technique. But certain yoga postures also help to reposition the solar plexus, and therefore cure many symptoms of IBS (see page 55). Other important elements of our treatment programme include adjustments to your diet to improve the function of the digestive system, and massage, which tones up the internal organs and relieves many symptoms of IBS.

diet   Adapting what and how you eat can help to reduce the severity of your symptoms, as follows:

• Eat varied foods according to their tastes. This is a yogic principle that has been practised successfully for thousands of years. Foods can be categorised according to their principal tastes: sweet, sour, pungent (spicy), insipid (watery), bitter, salty, astringent and so forth. You should aim to balance these tastes in your meals, as an excess of one type of food can cause digestive problems such as heartburn, bloating and diarrhoea. By varying your diet in this way, you will receive proper nutrition, balance your body's enzymes and also enhance the taste of your meals.

• Keep a note of any foods that trigger your IBS symptoms, and if necessary cut them out. Wheat or gluten products often cause bloating or diarrhoea, for example, and are therefore best avoided. Similarly, if you are intolerant to lactose (the natural sugar present in milk), avoid milk products. Another common IBS trigger is caffeine; this causes the bowel walls to tense up, which impairs the movement of food through the system and leads to constipation, abdominal cramps and poor digestion.

• Bitter foods are not consumed much in the West, but they can relieve certain symptoms of IBS. Bitter foods are alkaline, which can help to neutralise acids in the stomach; they also slow down the absorption of sugars. So those who experience a lot of heartburn, bloating and sluggish digestion, or who habitually eat a lot of sugary foods, should eat more bitter foods such as bitter gourd (karela), fenugreek leaves, courgettes, angostura bitters, unsweetened, flat tonic water and bitter lemon.

• Eat fewer citrus fruits, marinated foods, preserved (vinegary) foods, dry nuts and other products that can produce excess stomach acid. According to the principles of Yoga and Ayurveda, you should avoid excess sour or acid foods. The amount of acid in your stomach affects the part of your brain that controls appetite. So if you consume more acid, you force the body to eat more, creating an unwanted appetite which subsequently causes digestive problems. Moreover, excess stomach acid can neutralise the alkaline bile in the duodenum (part of the small intestine), which in turn can inhibit the finer digestion of protein, fats and carbohydrates. When this happens, the food sits there undigested for a long time, resulting in gas and bloating.

• For similar reasons, avoid very spicy meals because these can cause acidity or heartburn. This doesn't mean that you have to cut out spices altogether, just use them in moderation. Indeed, many herbs and spices have helpful remedial qualities: for example, turmeric has anti-inflammatory, antibacterial and anti acid properties, cumin can help relieve flatulence, garlic has antiseptic, deflatulent and cholesterol-regulating properties, chillies in moderation are energising and stress-relieving and ginger can treat nausea, low appetite and low energy and improve circulation.

• Avoid fermented and fungal products. These include yeast, bread, cheese (particularly blue cheeses), beer, mushrooms and yeast products (such as marmite and gravy granules). Mould-like fungi, however tasty they may be, are basically parasites: they have tentacles that penetrate into the gut lining, sucking the nutrients and producing gas and abdominal discomfort. Yeast or *Candida* can cause stomach cramps and diarrhoea – typical symptoms of IBS.

• Drinking lots of water is important to yogic practice. Fluids help to cleanse the body and certainly aid in eliminating stools, which is very useful. Always drink in-between meals, and have a glass of water 30–45 minutes after a meal. Avoid drinking too much during a meal: if you feel thirsty when you're eating, limit yourself to sipping water. This aids digestion, as the digestive juices are not diluted.

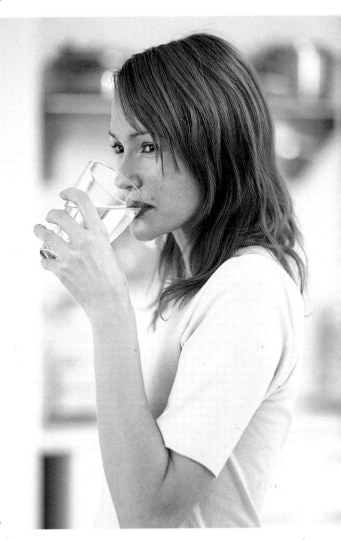

• Yogic principles place a lot of emphasis on cleansing the intestines from time to time to remove the by-products of digestion, stool masses, excess bile, acid and other secretions. Ideally, therefore, you should aim to go on a strict water or vegetable soup fast one day a week, consuming nothing but water or herbal teas containing cloves, liquorice, ginger and berries (particularly cranberries), or vegetable soup. If you find such a strict fast difficult to maintain, especially if you experience headaches or fluctuations in your mood, have a few glasses of carrot or apple juice during the day, a fruit salad for lunch, and end your fast in the evening with as much vegetable broth as you like.

• Plan your meals carefully. Breakfast should be substantial, consisting of grains (such as porridge or konji (a well-cooked soup of rice and vegetables), non-citrus fruits and sometimes protein (such as dried almonds soaked for 24 hours, a soft-boiled egg or some cottage cheese). Have enough lunch to fill about three-quarters of your stomach and base it on grains, protein such as fish, poultry or meat, and vegetables of all sorts of different tastes (for example, potatoes are starchy; aubergines, bland; yams, sharp; tomatoes, sour; okra, slimy; bitter gourd, bitter; radishes, very sharp; beetroot or turnips, sweet; and capsicums, pungent). Dinner should be light, easy to digest and eaten early, shortly after sunset; good foods at this time are fruits, rice, milk, soups, salads and lentils in various combinations.

• Eat slowly and chew well. Mastication turns food into a pulp, thus sparing the stomach from having to break it up itself by churning and secreting excess acid (which may cause heartburn, a major symptom of IBS). Food is best digested when it is broken into finer particles, which are then broken down further by enzymes before being absorbed. Eating slowly means that the enzymes in saliva can break carbohydrates up into sugars. These sugars send signals to the brain via the taste buds to say that food is on its way, which dampens your 'hunger pangs'. Thus you eat less and relieve the stomach of being forced to digest huge quantities of unchewed, dumped food. This will prevent indigestion and feelings of heaviness in the stomach – also symptoms of IBS.

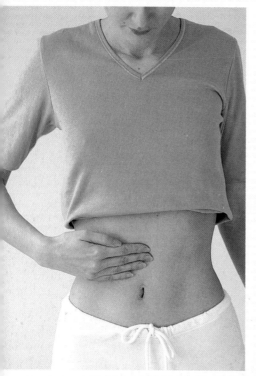

massage   A regular abdominal massage with sesame oil is very effective in toning up the intestines to improve peristalsis (the wave-like contractions of the walls of the digestive tract, which push food through the system). This helps to ease bowel movements and eliminate gas. The sesame oil warms up the tissues, improves circulation and tones up the abdominal muscles.

Abdominal massage is easy to perform yourself, and is best carried out first thing in the morning on an empty stomach. First lubricate the fingers and palm of one hand with the sesame oil and then begin to massage your abdomen in a clockwise movement, using your navel as the centre. Start with gentle pressure, and increase it gradually until you can feel the ascending, transverse and descending colon under your fingertips. Continue for 2 minutes or so.

Therapeutic postures

According to yogic science, most digestive disorders originate from a displacement of the navel or solar plexus (see page 51). All of the following exercises are designed to correct the position of the navel and thus help to prevent or treat IBS. Before you start, it's worth working through the Yoga Programme in Part 2 of the book (pages 35–47) to increase your spinal mobility. To benefit fully from the yoga poses, you should learn to control your breathing (see pages 32–34) so that you can perform them without straining other parts of your body. Always practise the Abdominal Lock on an empty stomach.

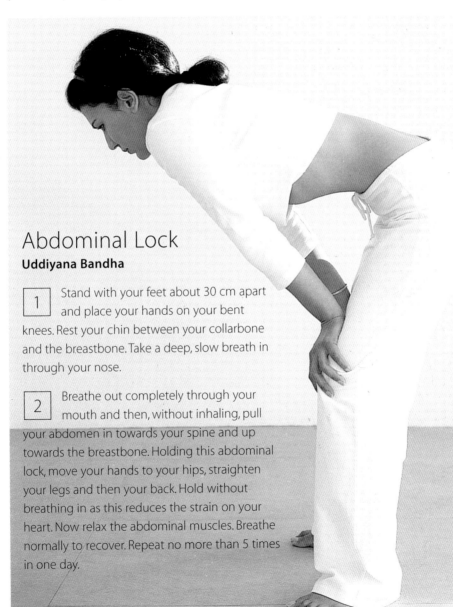

Abdominal Lock
Uddiyana Bandha

1. Stand with your feet about 30 cm apart and place your hands on your bent knees. Rest your chin between your collarbone and the breastbone. Take a deep, slow breath in through your nose.

2. Breathe out completely through your mouth and then, without inhaling, pull your abdomen in towards your spine and up towards the breastbone. Holding this abdominal lock, move your hands to your hips, straighten your legs and then your back. Hold without breathing in as this reduces the strain on your heart. Now relax the abdominal muscles. Breathe normally to recover. Repeat no more than 5 times in one day.

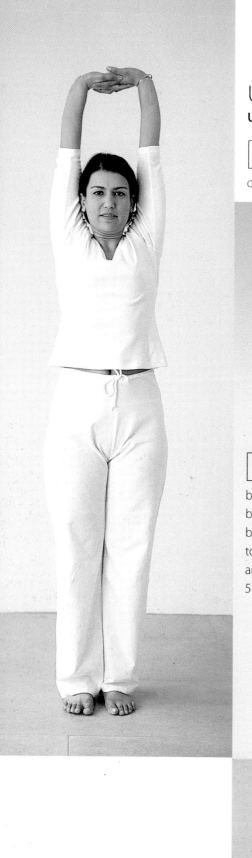

Upstretched Arms
Urdhva Hastottanasana

1. Stand with your feet slightly apart. Raise your arms above your head and interlock the fingers of your hands so that your palms are facing upwards.

2. Pull your arms back until they are by your ears and bend at the waist to the right. Then breathe out and straighten your body, pulling your stomach in towards your spine. Now breathe in and stretch down to the left. Repeat 5 times on each side.

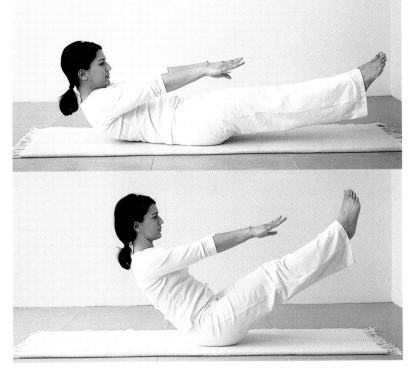

Boat Pose
Naukasana

1. Lie on your back with your legs stretched out, feet together, and your hands by the sides of your hips. Take a deep breath in and raise your head, legs and arms off the floor. Breathe out and lower your body to the floor, keeping your eyes level with your feet throughout. Rest. Repeat 5 times.

2. Once you are strong enough, try the full posture shown here. Keep your eyes level with your feet.

The Locust I
Shalabasana

1. Lie on your stomach with your arms stretched out in front and your forehead on the floor. Take a deep breath in and raise your right arm, left leg and head off the floor. Hold for 5 seconds, keeping your hips on the floor. Then breathe out and lower your forehead, arm and leg slowly to the floor. Rest. Repeat 5 times on each side.

2. When you are strong enough, raise both arms, legs and head off the floor. Keep your feet together or no more than hip-distance apart. Hold for 5 seconds. Then breathe out and lower your forehead, arms and legs slowly to the floor. Rest. Repeat 5 times. Over time, you may stay in the pose for 12 breaths before lowering your body to the floor.

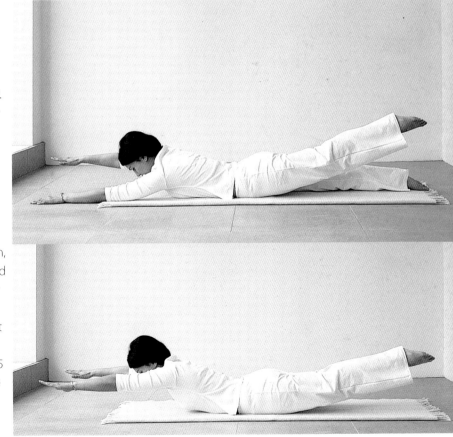

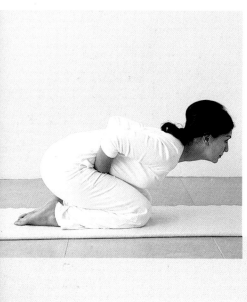

Frog Pose

Mandukasana

This posture is easily achieved by most people and is very good for relieving flatulence as any gases that have collected in the lower abdomen are forced out. The exercise very gently stretches the spine, enabling greater movement for all the abdominal organs.

1 Sit on your heels with your knees together and your palms pressed firmly one over the other on your abdomen near your navel. Bend forward, raising your head up a little for 5 breaths. Then sit up slowly on an in-breath. Breathe out and relax your shoulders, arms and facial muscles.

2 Now slowly lower your body to the floor behind you. If the stretch feels too strong in your thigh muscles, ease the tension out slowly and you will gradually be able to lower your body a bit more. Don't strain. Arch your back and interlock your hands underneath your head. Hold for 5–10 abdominal breaths and then return to the upright position.

3 Fold forward into the Child's Pose (see page 62) to relax your spine again before moving on.

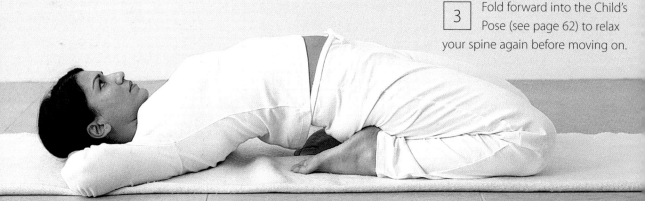

Abdominal Breathing

Pranayama

This gently massages your internal organs by moving the diaphragm, and relaxes the lower abdominal area, thereby improving the blood flow through the abdominal viscera and intestines.

1 Lie on your back. Relax your arms, legs, head and neck completely. Breathe in, extending your stomach completely like a balloon filled with air. Breathe out slowly and let the stomach relax. Don't try to pull in your stomach muscles at this stage. Repeat for at least 20 breaths.

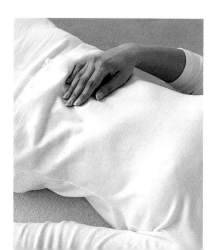

diabetes

Diabetes mellitus is a chronic condition in which the amount of sugar (glucose) in the blood is too high because the body is unable either to convert it into energy or to store it. Glucose is burned by the body's cells to make energy. Normally, a hormone called insulin, secreted by the pancreas, regulates the amount of glucose in the blood, but in people with diabetes either the body doesn't produce enough insulin (type I), or it is unable to use it properly (type II). Excess glucose then builds up in the blood, and is excreted through the urine.

High blood sugar has many complications. Firstly, it makes you feel tired, because even though there is plenty of glucose in the blood, your tissues (particularly your brain cells) can't use it without insulin. Then there is the constant thirst: you need to dilute all the sugar by drinking lots of water. And the more you drink, the more often you need to go to the toilet, especially at night, which can disturb your sleep. But the worst side-effect is that the glucose molecules can stick to the walls of the smaller blood vessels and clog them up. This can damage some of your organs, including the retina in your eyes, your heart muscles, nerves and kidneys, and may lead to male impotence and gangrene. In conventional medicine, the entire approach is to reduce the blood sugar and keep it under control. This can sometimes be managed with changes to the diet and lifestyle alone, but many people with diabetes have to take tablets or give themselves insulin injections. Our approach works through controlling the diet, increasing the body's metabolism through fairly strenuous yoga exercises, and increasing blood flow to the pancreas thanks to special postures.

diet   Your eating habits will have a huge impact on how well you manage to control your diabetes, and you should be given proper advice from your doctor or a nutritionist about avoiding all sugars and restricting to a minimum your intake of complex carbohydrates such as rice, pasta and bread. In addition, avoid excess fruits and alcohol. Herbal supplements – particularly the Ayurvedic ones containing bitter gourd (karela), fenugreek and jamuna (a fruit) – are useful as they help the formation of glucoproteids in the liver, which reduce excess sugar levels in the blood.

massage   The general massage routine described on pages 28–31, helps to improve circulation, even through tiny 'sugar-clogged' blood vessels in various parts of the body. A partner massage or a professional deep tissue massage once a week is very effective in overcoming muscle and brain fatigue and checking the complications of diabetes, which are mainly circulatory in origin. If you can't manage this, aim to massage yourself all over with sesame oil for about 10–15 minutes once or twice a week at bedtime, or an hour or so before a bath.

Therapeutic yoga

The postures in this section have several benefits: they improve blood flow to the pancreas, eyes and feet, helping to minimise the risk of such complications as poor eyesight or blurred vision and gangrene in the toes. They also boost the circulation in your smaller blood vessels and make for more economical absorption of oxygen, which helps to prevent heart, nerve and kidney damage. In addition to these poses, vigorous exercises such as brisk walking or cycling, when practised on a regular basis, are also invaluable as they increase your metabolic rate, which helps to burn the excess sugar in your blood.

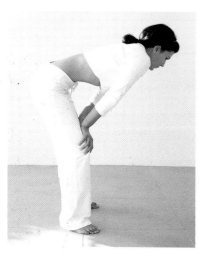

Abdominal Pump **Uddiyana Bandha**

This pumping action physically massages the pancreas, which is located in the upper part of the abdomen, and helps to improve circulation in the veins, thereby removing more impurities and toxins from the blood.

1 Stand with your feet apart. Bend forward with your hands on your knees. Take a deep breath in. Breathe out through your mouth, emptying your lungs.

2 Without inhaling, pull in your stomach and lift it up towards your ribcage. Hold for a count of 5, increasing this to 10 seconds over time. Let go and relax your breath. Repeat 5 times. Gradually, try to pump your stomach in and out 5 times without breathing in.

Forward Stretch

Paschimottanasana

By stretching the back of the thighs, this pose causes the abdominal wall to retract and compresses the abdominal viscera. This increases blood flow to the organs, facilitates the secretion of digestive juices and aids peristalsis.

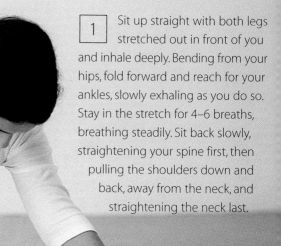

1 Sit up straight with both legs stretched out in front of you and inhale deeply. Bending from your hips, fold forward and reach for your ankles, slowly exhaling as you do so. Stay in the stretch for 4–6 breaths, breathing steadily. Sit back slowly, straightening your spine first, then pulling the shoulders down and back, away from the neck, and straightening the neck last.

Full Spinal Twist

Matsyendrasana

By twisting the upper spine, the upper digestive tract, pancreas and liver are decongested. This is very good for those with poor digestion, and the direct stimulation of the pancreas may encourage a release of insulin. If you are prone to cold hands and feet, this is an excellent posture as it improves the circulation in your extremities.

1 Sit with your left heel under your right buttock and place your right foot on the floor on the outside of your left knee. Practise sitting in this position for a few weeks before moving onto the next step.

2 Bring your left arm over your right knee and clasp your right ankle before placing your right hand on the floor behind you. Open out the front of your chest and look over your right shoulder. It is very important to keep the upper back straight. Breathe normally and hold the pose for 10 seconds. Repeat on the other side.

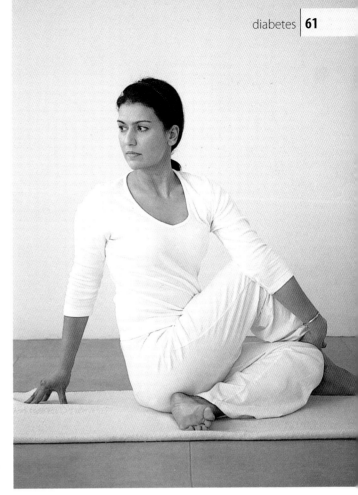

2 As you gain in experience, aim to reach further forwards, increasing the stretch over time until you can comfortably rest your head on your knees or shins. This will take a lot of careful practise to achieve.

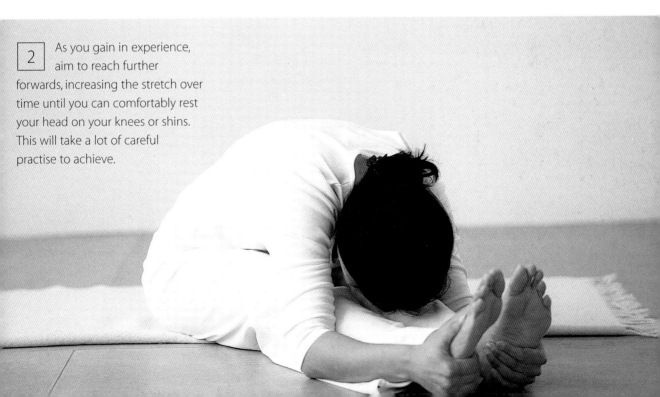

Crocodile Pose
Makarasana

1 Lie on your stomach with your forehead on the floor and stretch your arms forward with your palms together. Hold for 12 breaths.

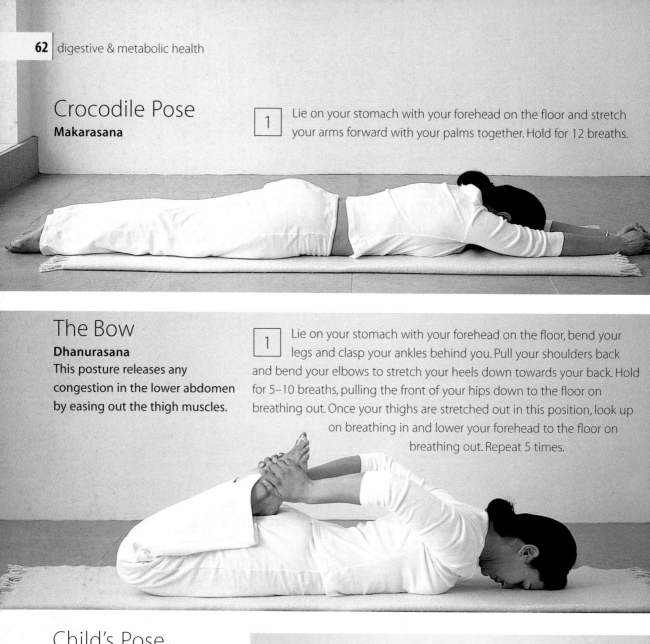

The Bow
Dhanurasana
This posture releases any congestion in the lower abdomen by easing out the thigh muscles.

1 Lie on your stomach with your forehead on the floor, bend your legs and clasp your ankles behind you. Pull your shoulders back and bend your elbows to stretch your heels down towards your back. Hold for 5–10 breaths, pulling the front of your hips down to the floor on breathing out. Once your thighs are stretched out in this position, look up on breathing in and lower your forehead to the floor on breathing out. Repeat 5 times.

Child's Pose
Balasana

1 Sit on your heels and bend forwards to place your forehead on the floor. Lower your arms by the sides of your legs and relax them. Feel your stomach against your thighs on breathing in and out. Try to press your buttocks slowly towards your heels by relaxing your whole body down to the floor. Relax the front of your hips, as well.

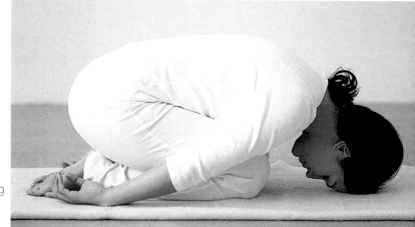

Neck Rolls
Griva Sakti Vikasaka

| 1 | Sit comfortably on a chair, on your heels or cross-legged on the floor. Lower your chin towards your chest and then rotate your neck slowly, first to the right and then to the left, breathing deeply. |

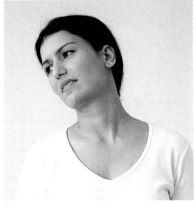

| 2 | Finish this by inhaling and lowering your chin to your sternum; hold your breath for at least 10 seconds. This is known as Jalandhara Bandha. Release slowly on exhaling, relaxing your shoulders. |

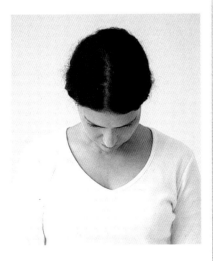

Corpse Pose
Shavasana

| 1 | Lie down on your back, with your neck straight. Take a deep breath in and stretch your arms up over your head, pointing your toes. Breathe out and release slowly. Repeat 5 times. |

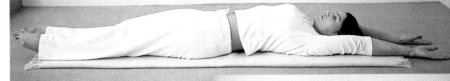

| 2 | Lower your arms. Breathe in and flex your toes while stretching your arms towards your feet. Exhale twice as slowly and relax. Repeat 5 times. |

| 3 | Now just relax in the Corpse Pose for at least 10 minutes, letting go of your body from your head to your toes and breathing at the abdomen. |

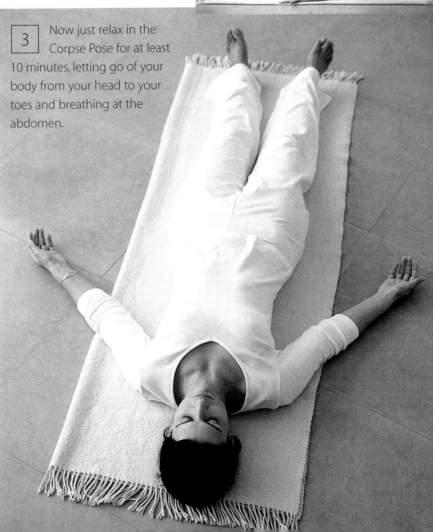

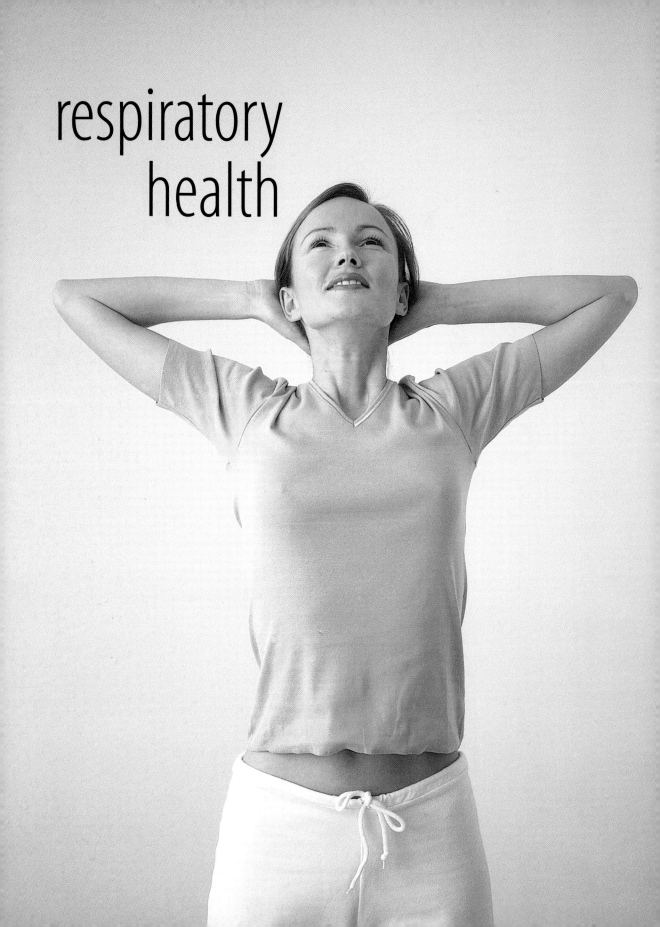

respiratory
health

asthma

This is usually an allergic condition in which the airways or bronchial tract go into spasm, obstructing the passage of air and causing shortness of breath and wheezing. During an asthma attack the muscles in the airways contract, narrowing the passages through which air can travel. Breathing in is fine, as the diaphragm is pulled down and the chest expands, making way for the air to come in. But breathing out through narrowed tubes is a great problem. This is why a wheeze or whistling sound occurs as the air is exhaled. Moreover, the cells in the airways produce more mucus than normal during an attack, which narrows the airways down further and makes breathing even more difficult.

Usually, asthma attacks are started by something that irritates your lungs; this is known as a trigger. Certain substances, called allergens, are well-known triggers, and include house dust mites, feathers, pollen and animal dander. If you breathe in something to which you are allergic, your body will try to protect itself from damage by expelling it. Your bronchial tract will constrict, you may start coughing, and the cells lining your airways will begin to secrete excess mucus to expel the allergen, all of which will set off an asthma attack. Other things can also act as triggers, including physical exertion, cold air, cigarette smoke and certain foods.

Asthma is normally treated with two types of medicines: bronchodilators, which help to relieve an attack by relaxing the airways and making it easier to breathe again; and anti-allergic remedies such as antihistamines and steroids which help to prevent attacks from occurring in the first place by working to keep your airways open all the time (through reducing inflammation and decreasing the mucus).

Our approach focuses on: avoiding known food allergens which might trigger an attack; neck and shoulder massage to increase blood flow to the pituitary gland (which controls all immunological processes in the body) and to improve sinus drainage and lymphatic drainage in the throat area; yoga postures and relaxation techniques to open up the chest area and facilitate breathing; and special breathing exercises to control attacks, expel excess phlegm or mucus and eliminate the phobia of breathlessness. The technique of holding your breath (see page 67, above) can really help to control acute asthma attacks, but needs to be practised several times a day to condition the mind during an actual episode.

diet   Some foods may act as triggers, provoking an asthma attack, so managing what you eat will help you to control the condition.

• Avoid mucus-producing substances like milk, cheese, ice cream, very spicy or fried food, bananas and excess carbohydrates, as the extra mucus will clog up your airways.

• Avoid all foods that cause allergies. Over a period of time, you'll learn what you are allergic to – dairy products, yeast, shellfish, nuts, monosodium glutamate (in Chinese foods), pineapples and citrus fruits are all common triggers.

• Limit foods that produce a lot of gas or flatulence such as yeast products, fizzy water and other carbonated drinks such as beer and champagne, citrus fruits, chickpeas, mushrooms and canned products. Abdominal gas raises the dome of the diaphragm and reduces the volume of the lungs, making them less functional.

• Eat carrots, non-citrus fruits and aim to include about 125 g of protein such as fish and chicken in your daily diet to ensure you receive balanced nutrition.

• If your child suffers from asthma, give him or her some highly nutritious marrow bone soup. You can prepare this by boiling marrow of lamb for 2 hours or so over a gentle heat with some vegetables. Use the stock over several days to make soup. This soup may sound a bit old-fashioned, but it contains lots of calcium, refined proteins and minerals which boost the body's natural healing powers and also help to prevent coughs and colds and therefore reduce the amount of mucus in the respiratory tract.

massage Try to follow the general sequence recommended on pages 28–31 as regularly as you can, paying particular attention to the throat area and the sinus points at the inner end of the eyebrows and below the cheek bones above the upper jaw. Gently massage the lymph nodes in the throat area (felt as glands) with Lifestyle Oil (see page 29) or Junior Massage Oil (100 ml apricot or grapeseed oil; 30 drops lavender; 20 drops eucalyptus) to help the lymph drain away, which decongests the sinuses and the upper respiratory tract. Then use your thumbs and fingers to work on the sensitive throat muscles and ligaments below the lower jaw.

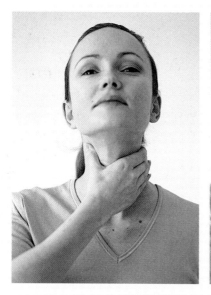
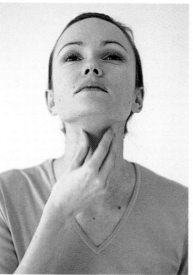
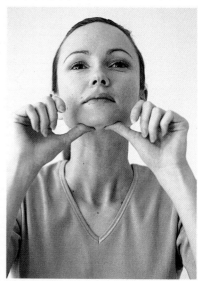

Breathing techniques

These are of huge importance in both the prevention and control of attacks. They will help you develop more regular, rhythmical breathing patterns without stress to the upper part of your chest. During an attack, try to practise retention breath. To do this, inhale for 3 seconds, hold your breath for 6–9 seconds, then exhale as slowly as possible. Continue to breathe slowly and deeply in this way for about 10 minutes, or until you feel the symptoms subsiding. This slows down your breathing and tricks your body into aborting the asthma attack by sending messages to the rest of the body to decongest the airways and dilate the lungs.

Abdominal Breathing

Pranayama

If your lung capacity is poor or you are unable to breathe deeply without experiencing a tightness in your chest or hyperventilating, this is the best breathing exercise to start with.

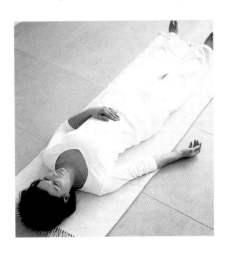

1   Lie down on your back and breathe at the stomach for 10 minutes. Let your stomach slowly rise up on breathing in and go down on breathing out. You shouldn't be using your chest at all. Just observe the ebb and flow of your breath.

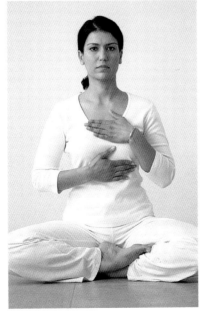

Complete Breath

Ujjayi Pranayama

1   Exhale completely, then fill your lungs slowly and steadily by relaxing the upper abdomen and expanding your chest. Try to make a hissing sound as you breathe by pressing your glottis against the top of your throat as you inhale and exhale.

2   Breathe out slowly. Try to make your out-breath slower than the in-breath. Aim for a ratio of 1:2 over time. Don't pull in your abdomen. Continue for 10 minutes.

3   Over time, start holding your breath for 5 seconds after inhaling, gradually increasing this to a ratio of 1:2:2. Repeat 20 such breaths. Your out-breath should still be twice as long as your in-breath. If you get out of breath, you are not yet ready for this step.

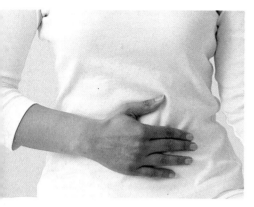

Cleansing Breath
Kapalabhati

Once you have mastered the first two breathing techniques, add the Kapalabhati in the mornings on an empty stomach. Remember, your out-breaths should be brief and active – you need to contract your abdominal muscles sharply to force the air out.

| 1 | Stand or sit comfortably. Straighten your upper back and pull your shoulders back. Close your mouth and look straight ahead. Breathe in fully through your nose. Now breathe out quickly, pulling your stomach in. Pause between breaths for a second or so, and then breathe in again, taking your time. Repeat 25 times.

Bellows Breath
Bhastrika

In this technique the in- and out-breaths are quick and forceful like the bellows of a blacksmith. Your navel should relax on breathing in and pull in sharply on breathing out. You may feel slightly dizzy to begin with or want to cough. If you are breathless, or your chest tightens up, you are probably using the upper chest or pulling in and relaxing your navel the wrong way round, so go back to Kapalabhati.

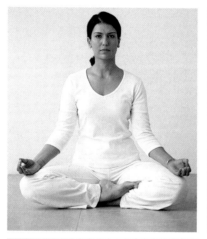
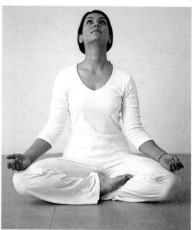

| 1 | Stand or sit comfortably with a straight spine and your shoulders back. Look straight ahead and close your mouth. Take a deep breath in through your nose and relax your stomach. Breathe out forcefully, as if you were sniffing out, and pull in your upper abdomen. Keep repeating in a continuous series of 25 quick, forceful pumpings.

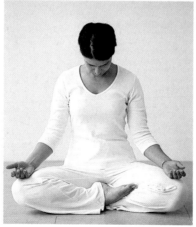
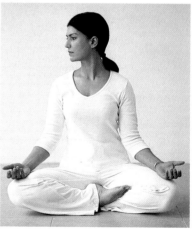

| 2 | Repeat with your shoulders pulled back, your chest forwards and looking up to stretch the front of your neck.

| 3 | Perform a further 25 pumpings with your chin down towards your chest, focusing on the area below your ribcage.

| 4 | Repeat, looking alternately over each shoulder: exhale as you turn your head to the side and inhale coming back to centre.

Therapeutic postures

Try to work through the following exercises on a regular basis. When you are familiar with these postures, gradually start to include the exercises from the Yoga Programme in the Healthy Living Routine (pages 35–47).

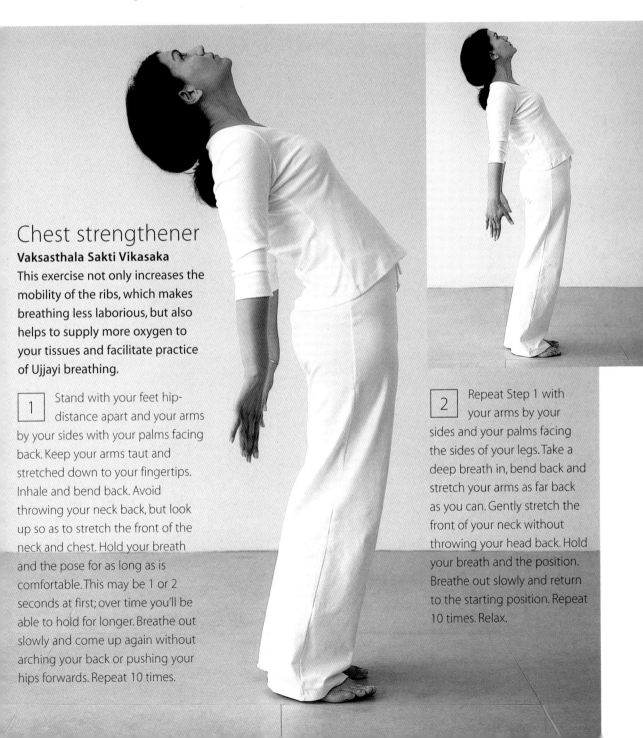

Chest strengthener
Vaksasthala Sakti Vikasaka
This exercise not only increases the mobility of the ribs, which makes breathing less laborious, but also helps to supply more oxygen to your tissues and facilitate practice of Ujjayi breathing.

1 Stand with your feet hip-distance apart and your arms by your sides with your palms facing back. Keep your arms taut and stretched down to your fingertips. Inhale and bend back. Avoid throwing your neck back, but look up so as to stretch the front of the neck and chest. Hold your breath and the pose for as long as is comfortable. This may be 1 or 2 seconds at first; over time you'll be able to hold for longer. Breathe out slowly and come up again without arching your back or pushing your hips forwards. Repeat 10 times.

2 Repeat Step 1 with your arms by your sides and your palms facing the sides of your legs. Take a deep breath in, bend back and stretch your arms as far back as you can. Gently stretch the front of your neck without throwing your head back. Hold your breath and the position. Breathe out slowly and return to the starting position. Repeat 10 times. Relax.

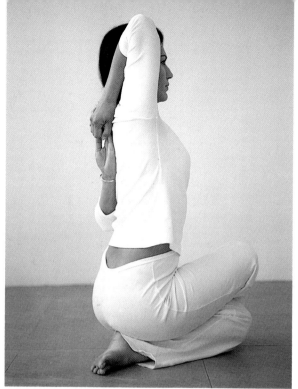

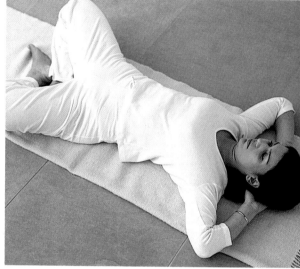

Cow Pose

Gomukhasana

This asana can help to treat many lung conditions. Since one lung cannot be expanded efficiently in this position, the other has to work more vigorously, which opens up and cleanses innumerable pores and alveoli (air sacs). You then swap sides to work the second lung. If you feel a slight strain in the lower back you may have arched it too much, so lie in the Child's Pose for a minute or two to relax the lower back (see page 62).

1 Sit on the floor with your legs in front of you. Now bend your left leg so that your heel is under your buttock. Bend your right leg and cross it over your left knee so that both knees are in line, your right heel towards left hip. (Don't worry if you can't get into this position – sit on a chair or stand instead.)

2 Bend your left arm up behind your back and raise your right arm. Now bend your right arm down at the elbow and try to clasp your hands behind your back. Aim to interlock your fingers over time. Remain in the position for 5–10 breaths and breathe normally. Repeat, reversing positions by sitting on your right heel and lifting up your left arm.

Fish Pose I

Matsyasana

This relaxing posture is particularly good for asthma because, by putting your hands under your head, you expand your thorax and open up your lungs.

1 Lie on your back with your hands under your head, and cross your legs, pulling your ankles as close as is comfortable to your body. Breathe deeply and comfortably for at least 1 minute. Keep your entire spine relaxed towards the floor. Now relax your breath. You will find yourself breathing naturally with the abdomen as the diaphragm is freed in this posture. It goes down on inhaling, making your stomach rise, and goes up on exhaling, so your stomach relaxes inwards.

Relaxing meditation

If you suffer from asthma, you will benefit hugely from learning how to meditate. Not only does meditation help to reduce anxiety, but numerous studies have shown that it also relaxes the bronchial tract, thus clearing the airways. In the long term, it may alleviate the condition altogether. You'll find advice on how to meditate on pages 20–21.

sinusitis and catarrh

There are four pairs of air-filled cavities, known as sinuses, around the nose and ears, which are connected by narrow channels to the back of the nose. These air-filled chambers help to decrease the weight of the head and give acoustic value to the voice. The sinuses are lined with a membrane which secretes mucus to keep the nasal tract moist. Under normal circumstances this mucus drains away naturally, keeping air circulating around the sinuses. But if the sinuses become inflamed – in a condition called sinusitis – the channels between the sinuses and the nasal cavity will be blocked and mucus can accumulate in the cavities, causing pain, congestion and breathing difficulties, loss of smell and sensitivity to light.

Acute sinusitis lasts for approximately three weeks and can be caused by: viral infections; an acute chill when the head is exposed to extreme cold air (for example, going out with wet hair on a cold day with a blistering wind); acute constipation, which probably causes toxins in the bowels to be secreted via mucus into the cavities of the sinuses; an allergic reaction; and consumption of mucus-producing substances (see overleaf).

Chronic sinusitis lasts for much longer, and occurs when the causes of the sinusitis themselves become chronic. For example, long-term digestive problems such as chronic heartburn, diarrhoea, flatulence and constipation can result in chronic sinusitis as the toxins resulting from impaired digestion are secreted through excess mucus in the sinuses.

Blocked sinuses are breeding grounds for anaerobic bacteria, which thrive without oxygen. But as soon as air is pumped back into the sinuses, the bacteria die and the sinus infection is cleared, so there is no real need for antibiotics. Our treatment concentrates on reducing the amount of mucus in the sinuses (through your diet and cleansing techniques) and breathing exercises to get air circulating properly. As a preventative measure, avoid sudden exposure to cold water or air.

Catarrh is an acute inflammation of the mucous membrane of the upper respiratory tract, including the sinuses, nose, throat, trachea and even the eyes and the ears. When the body is run down, opportunistic germs and viruses in the air lodge on the lining of the mucous membrane. The body begins to produce copious amounts of mucus to wash off the viruses or germs, hence the watery discharges. If the immune system doesn't manage to eliminate the invading organisms within 36–48 hours of the attack, the germs enter the cells of the mucous membrane and cause inflammation. The lining thickens, resulting in a blocked nose, sinusitis and a sore throat, as well as the discharge of a thick, yellowish-green mucus. Fever, all-over aches and pains, extreme fatigue and headache may also occur.

The fever is a defensive reaction. Germs and viruses thrive well at optimum body temperature, so the body raises its temperature to provide a less favourable environment for the germs or virus to multiply. Instead of taking medicaments such as paracetamol to lower the fever, use a fan or turn on the air-conditioning (if you have it) to lower the room temperature, apply cold packs (towels dipped in cold water) to the forehead and the abdomen, and dress lightly to aid the body from raising the fever beyond 40°C.

diet *Sinusitis:* Avoid ice cold water, ice, cheese and dairy foods in general, mushrooms, yeast, excess chocolate or sweets, spicy foods and canned products as these may exacerbate the amount of mucus in your sinuses. Be sure to keep drinking plenty of water, so as to avoid constipation, but don't drink it too cold – warm water is best. Similarly, stay clear of all chilled drinks and ice cream. Other foods to avoid are: cheese, milk, yoghurt, cream, butter, citrus fruits, red meat, fried food, very spicy dishes,

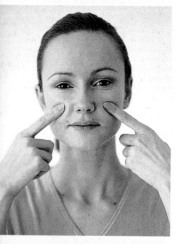

preserved foods and fermented foods (such as beer, yeast products and vinegar). If you are suffering from acute sinusitis, spend a couple of days eating non-citrus fruits and vegetable broth, all washed down with lots of warm water, to help eliminate the toxins and reduce the mucus discharge. *Catarrh:* Drink warm water infused with ginger and some honey to dry up the mucus. Another good dish for catarrh sufferers is a soup made from onion, garlic, ginger, black pepper and fresh chicken stock; these ingredients are hot from a macrobiotic point of view, which helps to eliminate colds and catarrh problems.

massage Mix up a special Sinus Oil from 4 parts mustard oil and 3–4 parts organic, cold-pressed sesame oil. Then place 2 drops of this oil into each nostril, twice daily. This loosens up the mucus, helping to clear the sinuses, and also coats the lining of the airways, preventing other particles from causing irritation.

The neck and spine massage described on page 29 helps to overcome the fatigue caused by tensed muscles in the neck. Fatigue weakens the immune system and makes the body more susceptible to colds and allergic reactions. To help relieve the symptoms of congestion, press the sinus points on the cheeks and on the inside of each eyebrow, as shown on the left.

Therapeutic poses

The exercises on the next three pages assist directly with draining your sinuses and dislodging mucus from the chest, helping to decongest your airways and to provide immediate relief from the unpleasant symptoms of sinusitis and catarrh. You should also follow the sequences recommended for backache and neck pain (see pages 88–90 and 93–100) as these increase blood flow to your facial muscles and unblock the channels for draining the sinuses. Try to maintain a good stretch in your spine, neck and shoulders, although you may experience some discomfort in your sinuses and forehead when you lower your head in some of the forward stretches, or when placing your head on the floor. This is due to the sudden build-up of pressure from increased blood flow to the head.

Nasal Douche
Jal Neti

This isn't strictly speaking a yoga pose, but a Kriya or cleansing process. The salt solution helps to dissolve away any secretions or deposits from inhaled air, thereby releasing any mucus. It also increases the circulation of blood in all the tissues around the sinuses, while the cleansing effects benefit the eyes and nasal passages as well.

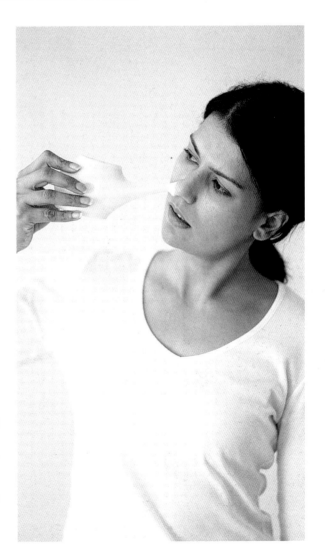

1 Fill a pot with a spout with about two glasses of warm water and add a teaspoon of salt. Place the spout into your right nostril by tilting your head to the side. Water should begin to flow through the nostril and out through the other. Breathe through your mouth throughout this exercise, otherwise water will enter the upper part of your nasal passage, creating discomfort in the sinuses. Refill the pot and repeat with the left nostril.

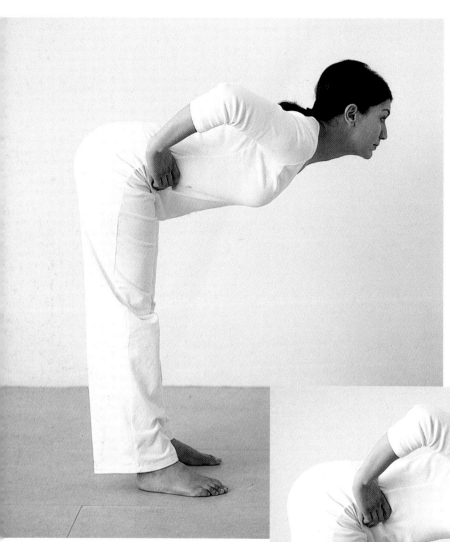

Bellows Breath
Bhastrika

This version of Bhastrika is done leaning forwards rather than standing upright in order to clear any water still remaining in the nostrils after the Nasal Douche.

1 In a standing position, place your hands on your hips and bend forward at an angle of 90°. Bend your knees slightly if you are stiff or have a sore back. Close your mouth and keep your eyes open. Take a deep breath in through your nose and allow your stomach to relax. Breathe out forcefully, as though you were sniffing out, and actively pull in your diaphragm.

2 Keep breathing in and out quickly through the nostrils in a continuous series of 25 quick, forceful pumpings. Turn your head right, left, up and down for one breath in each direction.

3 Finish by lying down to relax in the Corpse Pose (see pages 46–47). Pay particular attention to relaxing and stretching your neck.

Lion Pose

Simhasana

This has an unrivalled ability to dislodge catarrh from the upper respiratory tract. It is usually done on your heels with your hands on your thighs, but you can stand over a sink (in case you want to spit out any catarrh released) or sit on a chair if you prefer. Omit this posture if you've got high blood pressure.

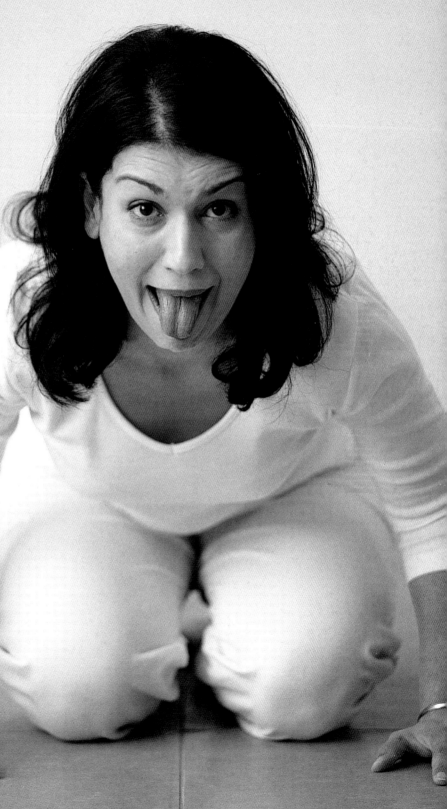

| 1 | Breathe in and stick your tongue out as far as possible. Tighten your facial muscles and look fierce. Lean forwards and tense up your arms and hands like claws. Your neck should also be taut. Keeping your tongue stuck out, breathe out ferociously at the base of your throat. Sit back, straighten your neck and relax your arms. Repeat 2–3 times only, relaxing your breath in-between. If your throat is weak this posture can cause soreness, so don't repeat it too often in one session. |

| 2 | Now lie down and relax in the Corpse Pose (see pages 46–47). |

bone & muscle health

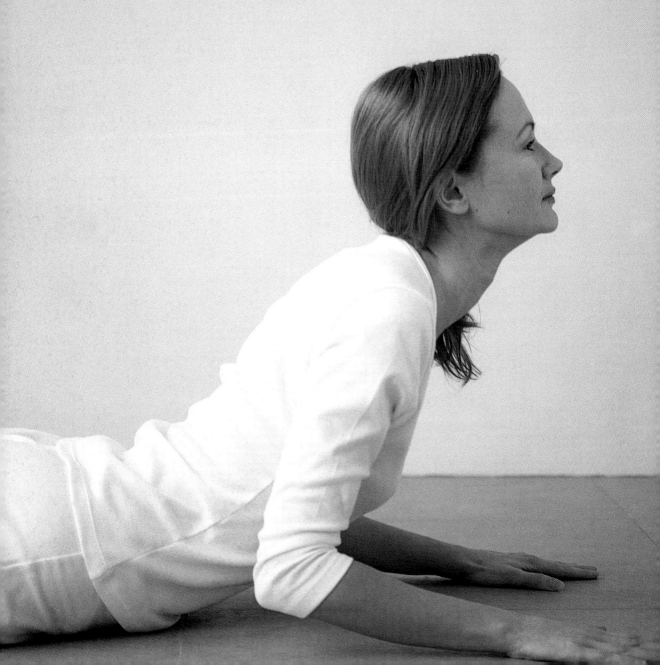

arthritis

Joints are formed where two or more bones meet, and allow your body to bend and turn in all sorts of different ways. They are designed to make movement as fluid and easy as possible. The ends of the bones are lined with a smooth tissue called cartilage which prevents friction, and surrounded by a lubricating fluid (known as synovial fluid). But despite this protection, your joints are delicate and susceptible to wear and tear, and as you age you may become more prone to one of a number of conditions known collectively as arthritis.

The word arthritis refers to a number of inflammatory conditions that cause pain, swelling and stiffness in the joints. There are many different types of arthritis, including osteoarthritis, rheumatoid arthritis, gout and reactive arthritis.

Osteoarthritis is the most common form of the disease, and is characterised by the gradual wearing away of the protective cartilage that covers the ends of the bones within the joint. If the bone underneath is exposed, outgrowths of new bone (called osteophytes) may form, which lead to pain and reduced mobility. The tissue surrounding the joint can also become inflamed, which causes fluid to accumulate, resulting in swelling and pain. Osteoarthritis most often affects weight-bearing joints such as the spine, hips, knees and ankles and is thought to be caused by general wear and tear. In our opinion, it is the weakening of the weight- and stress-bearing muscles – the body's shock absorbers – that is responsible for damaging the cartilage and membrane that surrounds the joints. These muscles should absorb the impact when, say, you jump down from a height, and prevent the surfaces within your hip, knee and ankle joints from colliding with each other. But if they become weak, they could actually increase the strain on your joints. For example, weakness of the spinal muscles and quadriceps muscles in your thighs may lead to extra pressure on your hip and knee joints, especially when you are walking and climbing stairs. Exercises to strengthen your muscles and improve the mobility of your joints therefore play a very important role in helping to prevent and treat osteoarthritis. Treatment should also aim to prevent further degeneration of the joint surfaces, and – if the joints are properly protected and treated – to rectify any damage already done.

Rheumatoid arthritis is an autoimmune disease in which the body mistakenly identifies its own joint tissue as foreign and produces antibodies to attack it. This aggressive onslaught immobilises the joints and results in swelling, pain, stiffness, and sometimes permanent damage or deformity. The disorder can affect joints throughout the body, and often appears first in the smaller joints of the hands and feet. Treatment with anti-inflammatory creams or a massage with Ayurvedic oils may help to control some of the symptoms, but it won't bring long-term relief. Instead, the

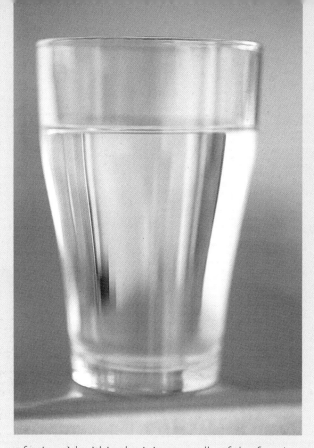

approach has to be general, directed towards the whole body, so that the immune system calms down. Steroids, anti-inflammatory drugs, immuno-suppressants and painkillers will have a limited effect, even in the long term, so diet, massage and gentle exercise are crucial. Individual joints are often too angry or inflamed to be exercised, so our recommendations for therapeutic yoga focus on your general wellbeing.

Gout is a form of arthritis caused by crystalline deposits of uric acid within the joints, usually of the feet. It occurs when the kidneys stop excreting uric acid (a by-product of the breakdown of proteins) properly. Uric acid then accumulates in the blood and crystallises on the surfaces of the joint, forming deposits which tear the synovial membrane encasing the joint, causing acute inflammation. The affected joint then becomes red, hot, swollen, stiff, and very painful. Anti-inflammatory drugs and uric-acid-eliminating drugs such as allupurinol help to control the condition, but the best treatment is prevention, so your diet is especially important (see below).

diet Excess blood sugar, cholesterol and uric acid are known to cause inflammation and pain in your joints. To prevent these substances from building up in your body, limit your intake of chocolate, cakes, sugar, fatty or fried foods, butter, cheese, red meat, offal and shellfish. Similarly, dairy products, citrus fruits (which produce excess stomach acid), spicy foods, nuts, white wine, vinegar and smoking can also make the joint surfaces sensitive, so don't overindulge in these. Deficiencies of certain minerals – particularly calcium and magnesium – cause joint pain as the cartilage or bone gets slightly brittle; supplements are therefore highly recommended. Prolonged constipation inhibits the absorption of calcium, so take steps to avoid this condition by eating papaya, prunes, figs, beetroot and spinach, and be sure to drink 1.5 litres of water a day. If you are prone to gout, avoid red meat, shellfish, cheese, offal, alcohol, kidney beans and tomatoes, which contain a lot of purines (by-products of protein metabolism that are deposited on the joints as uric acid crystals, causing inflammation).

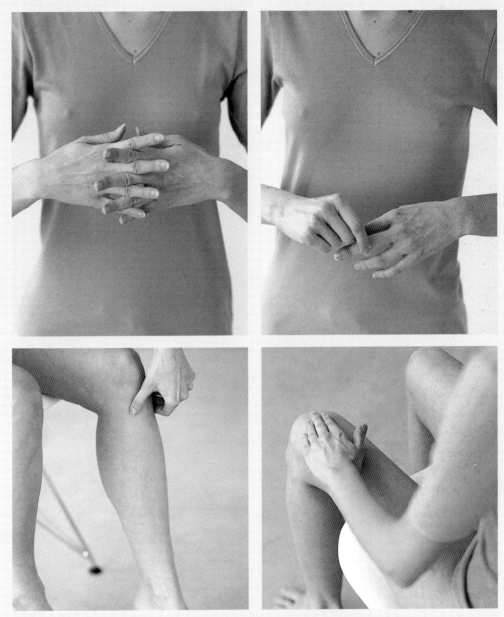

massage Using some special Joint Oil (100 ml Ayurvedic Mahanarayan oil, 5 ml clove oil and 1 ml wintergreen oil), lubricate your hands and then massage the muscles and ligaments above and below the affected joints, stroking downwards. Work on the ligaments that bind the affected joint, focusing on the areas that are most sensitive. If possible, get someone else to massage you: some areas will initially be quite sore and you won't want to hurt yourself, whereas a friend, partner or professional massage therapist is likely to be a bit firmer. You'll find that as the treatment takes hold, the pain eases remarkably, often at the end of the session.

Therapeutic postures

The following yoga poses are strongly advised for generally loosening up the main joints and for strengthening the back. Most of the exercises suggest you begin by standing up with your feet slightly apart; as your body strengthens and stabilises, try starting with your feet together.

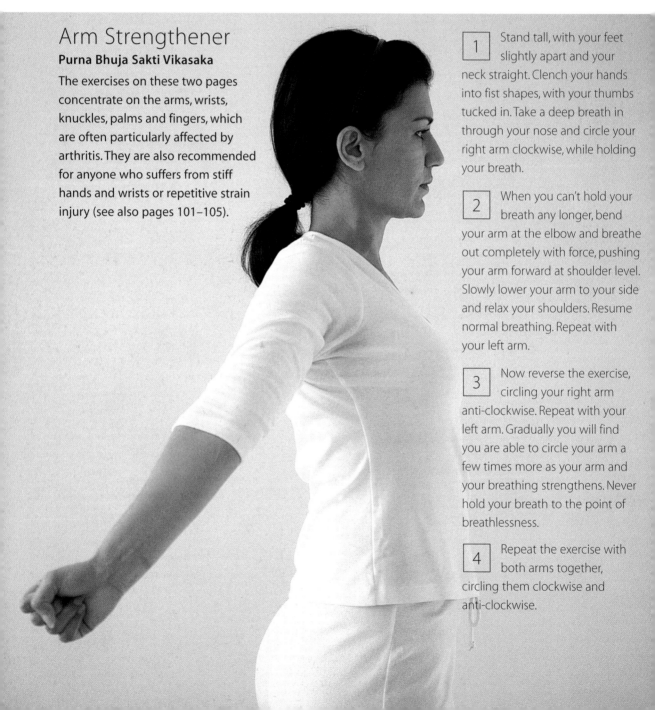

Arm Strengthener
Purna Bhuja Sakti Vikasaka

The exercises on these two pages concentrate on the arms, wrists, knuckles, palms and fingers, which are often particularly affected by arthritis. They are also recommended for anyone who suffers from stiff hands and wrists or repetitive strain injury (see also pages 101–105).

1 Stand tall, with your feet slightly apart and your neck straight. Clench your hands into fist shapes, with your thumbs tucked in. Take a deep breath in through your nose and circle your right arm clockwise, while holding your breath.

2 When you can't hold your breath any longer, bend your arm at the elbow and breathe out completely with force, pushing your arm forward at shoulder level. Slowly lower your arm to your side and relax your shoulders. Resume normal breathing. Repeat with your left arm.

3 Now reverse the exercise, circling your right arm anti-clockwise. Repeat with your left arm. Gradually you will find you are able to circle your arm a few times more as your arm and your breathing strengthens. Never hold your breath to the point of breathlessness.

4 Repeat the exercise with both arms together, circling them clockwise and anti-clockwise.

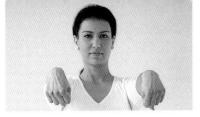

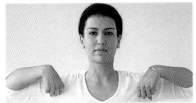

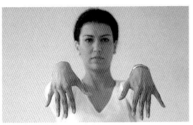

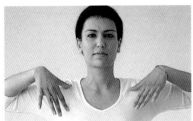

Finger Strengthener
Anguli Sakti Vikasaka

1 Stretch your arms out in front of you at shoulder level, with your fingers bent at the joints to create a claw-like effect.

2 Stiffen both arms from your shoulders to fingertips, and slowly bend them back at the elbow; they should tremble with the effort. Imagine some resistance to your movements. Repeat 5 times.

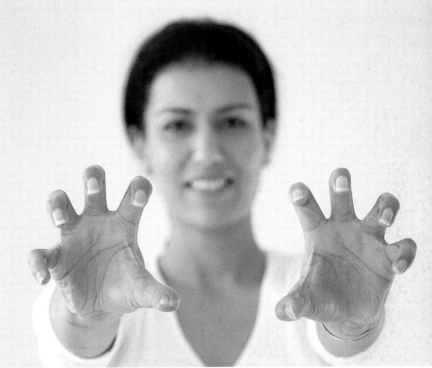

Wrist Strengthener
Mani Bandha Sakti Vikasaka

1 Standing tall, stretch your arms out in front at shoulder level, your fists loosely clenched. Keeping your arms strong and still, move your wrists up and down as far as they will go. Repeat 5 times.

2 Bend your arms and clench your fists up by your shoulders, your palms facing out. Again, firmly move your wrists up and down, repeating 5 times.

3 Now repeat Step 1 with your hands open and your palms facing down.

4 Finally, repeat Step 2 with your fingers spread wide.

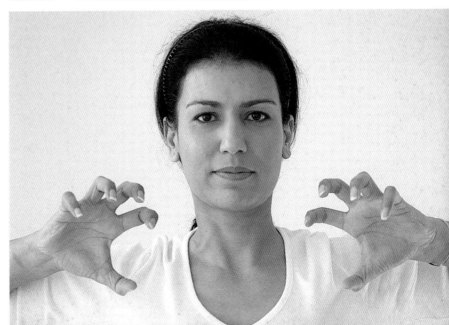

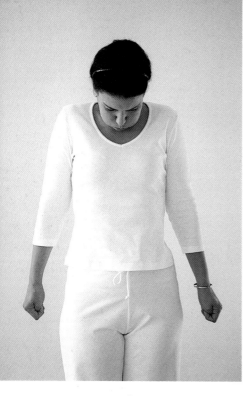

Shoulder Strengthener

Bahu Mula Sakti Vikasaka

This exercise helps to loosen up the arms, shoulders and neck, as well as to strengthen the shoulder joints and shoulder blades.

1 Stand tall with your arms by your sides and your feet slightly apart. Loosely clench your fists and tuck your thumbs in. Suck in air through your mouth until your cheeks are puffed out, and then hold your breath (unless you have high blood pressure, in which case breathe normally throughout). Lower your chin to rest on your sternum.

2 Still holding your breath, quickly move your shoulders up and down, keeping your stiffened arms by your sides. When you can no longer comfortably hold your breath, exhale slowly through your nose and straighten your neck, relaxing your arms, shoulders and hands. Relax your breath. Repeat 5 times.

Leg and Foot Strengthener

Pada Mula Sakti Vikasaka

1 Stand with your feet together, your body straight and relaxed. Breathe in and come up onto your toes, then lower your heels up and down in a spring-like motion. Repeat 25 times.

2 Stand with your feet at least 45 cm apart and place your hands on your hips. Breathe in and bend the right knee, transferring your body weight onto your right leg. Breathe out and straighten the leg. Repeat on the left side. Keep swaying from right to left in this way 25 times on each side.

3 Stand straight. Lift your left foot about 25 cm off the floor in front of you. Keeping the leg straight, circle your ankle clockwise and then anti-clockwise. This loosens and strengthens stiff ankles. If you find balancing difficult, you can perform this exercise sitting on a chair. Repeat 5 times with each leg, working up to 10 times.

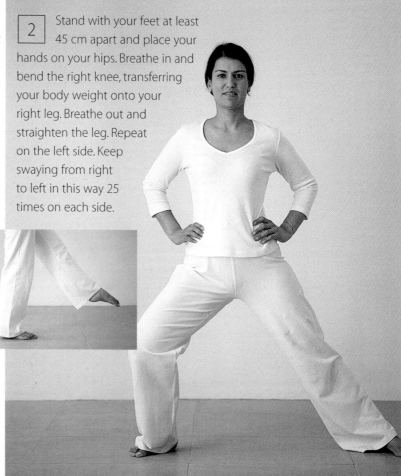

Heel Raise
Jangha Sakti Vikasaka

1 | Lie on your back, with your feet hip-distance apart and your knees bent. Press your chin down towards your neck and relax your shoulders. Pull your spine towards the floor; breathe normally.

2 | Raise your right foot about 20 cm off the floor, without extending the knee, and then lower the heel to the floor once more. Repeat this movement quickly, working up to about 25 times on each leg. Keep your lower back firmly against the floor and be careful not to move your knees from the starting position.

Supine Chair
Supta Jangha

1 | Lie down on your back, facing a wall, with your arms by your sides and your neck straight. Bend your knees, keeping your feet on the floor. Breathe in, raise your right foot and press it against the wall. Hold for a count of 10. Breathe out and lower your foot to the floor. Now swap legs. Repeat 5 times on each side. On finishing, stretch out both legs for 5–12 breaths. Bend your knees and lower your feet to the floor.

Squatting

Utktasana

The exercises you have just done improve the strength of your muscles. When you are ready, try the following postures, which will increase the stability of your joints.

1 Stand with your feet slightly apart and stretch your arms out in front of you. Take a deep breath in and bend your knees gradually until your thighs are parallel to the floor – as if you were sitting in a chair. Keep your heels and toes on the floor at all times, and your knees bent over your toes. Breathe out and stand up slowly. Repeat 5 times.

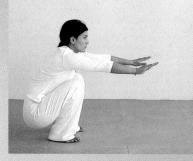

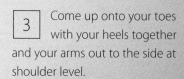

2 When your back and thigh muscles are strong enough, you can try the full posture by lowering yourself all the way down, until your buttocks are just off the floor. Repeat 5 times and then return to a standing position.

3 Come up onto your toes with your heels together and your arms out to the side at shoulder level.

4 Keeping your spine erect, breathe in and bend your knees over your toes. Hold for a count of 5. Breathe out, straighten your legs, flatten your feet and relax your arms. Repeat 5 times.

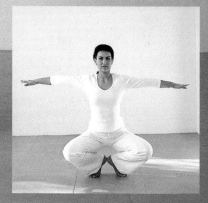

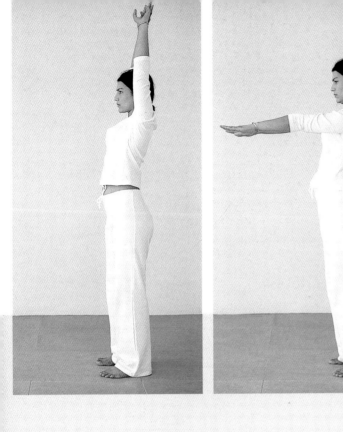

The Crow
Kakasana

1. Stand with your feet slightly apart. Take a deep breath in and raise your arms, stretching up to the ceiling.

2. Breathe out, come up onto your toes and lower your arms in front of you to shoulder level.

3. Keeping your back straight, bend your knees and place your hands on the floor between your thighs. Breathe normally, rocking on your toes with your head down towards the floor. Breathe in and stand up. Stretch your arms up and come down again on breathing out. Repeat 5 times.

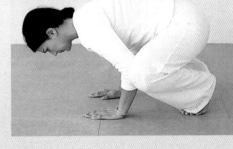

4. If you can, transfer your body weight onto your wrists and finger joints and relax your neck. Then lift your feet off the floor slightly. You may bend the elbows against the insides of the knees at this stage to support the posture. Hold the position for as long as is comfortable. Repeat once only.

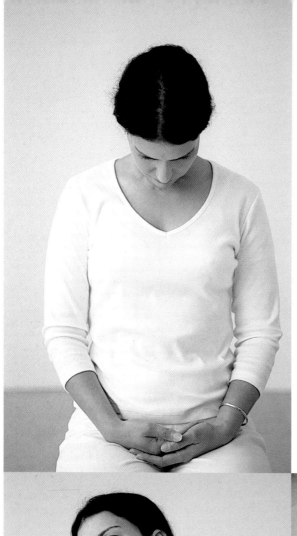

Neck Rolls

Griva Sakti Vikasaka

These neck rolls gently stretch out the front and back of your shoulders without aggravating your neck joints.

1. Sit comfortably on a chair, on your heels or cross-legged on the floor. Lower your chin towards your chest bone.

2. Rotate your neck slowly, first to the right and then to the left, breathing deeply throughout. Repeat 10 times.

3. Finish the session by lying down in the Corpse Pose (see pages 46–47). Relax.

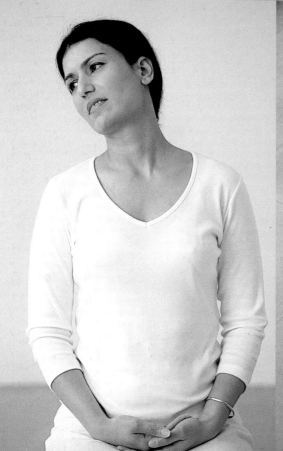

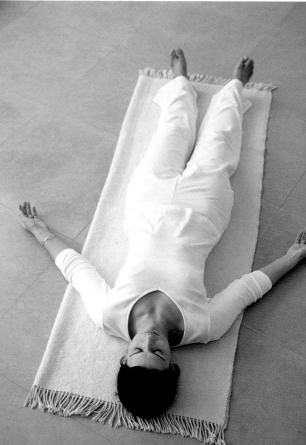

neck pain

Forming the top part of the spine, the neck consists of 7 vertebrae and 14 joints which allow the head to move in all directions. The more mobile a part of the body is, however, the more fragile it is. Thus the neck is prone to dislocations and other traumas.

Anatomically, the neck has a very complex structure. Besides housing the thick spinal cord and all the nerves for the upper part of the body, it has a pair of arteries known as the vertebral arteries which effectively supply the entire subconscious part of the brain. So an injury to the neck, such as whiplash, may not only cause physical problems such as tingling, pain and numbness, due to joint and nerve damage, but also other problems – including fatigue, headaches, dizziness, loss of balance, panic attacks, disrupted hormonal cycles and sleep disturbances – which result from reduced blood flow through the vertebral arteries to the subconscious brain.

Over the past 20 years, we have studied the role of the vertebral arteries in a whole range of neurological, emotional, hormonal and immunological conditions and discovered that a specially developed deep massage of the ligaments, muscles, tendons and joints of the neck – known as the Ali Technique – followed by therapeutic yoga, can help to relieve many of these health problems by improving blood flow through the vertebral arteries.

diet Acid foods affect the collagen in your ligaments, causing them to weaken, so avoid citrus fruits such as lemons, oranges and grapefruits, white wine, champagne, pineapple, tomatoes and also spicy foods. Instead, concentrate on eating potassium-rich foods such as carrots, which tone up your muscles, protein such as eggs, fish and chicken to help build up your muscles, calcium to strengthen your bones, and plenty of fresh non-citrus fruits. Avoid coffee and salt as these cause your muscles to tense up, and excess alcohol, which dehydrates your muscles.

massage Ideally, if you are having neck problems, we recommend that you consult a doctor or massage therapist familiar with the Ali Technique. A 10-minute self-massage, however, can also be very effective. Massage the area from one ear lobe to the other with your thumbs and fingers. You may find that this feels a bit tender; this is because tight neck muscles can create tension. Then use your thumbs and fingers to massage either side of the neck, focusing on both the superficial and the deeper muscles. Again, this might be a bit painful, particularly if you have a desk job or use a computer a lot, as these muscles can get overstrained. Then move on to the shoulders and upper back.

Therapeutic postures

This sequence of exercises is essential for stress management and your general wellbeing as they loosen the neck muscles and improve blood flow to the brain.

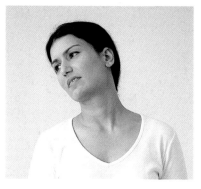

Neck Strengthener
Griva Sakti Vikasaka

1 Sit or stand upright with your back straight and your mouth closed. Lower your chin to the front of your neck. Rotate your head in a semi-circle from left to right and back again. Do this slowly with deep, slow breaths, so as to feel all the muscles in your upper back and the side of your neck stretching out, releasing tension in the jaw. The aim is to touch your shoulder with your ear, without raising your shoulder – relax your shoulders throughout. Repeat 5 times.

2 Interlock your fingers and place your palms at the nape of your neck. Breathe in and open out your elbows to the sides as you lower your chin to the front of your neck.

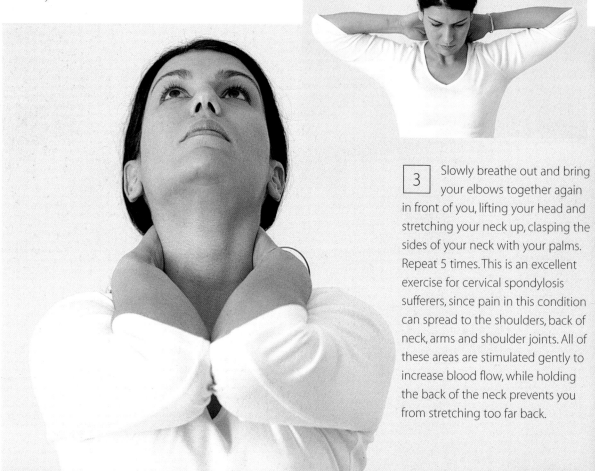

3 Slowly breathe out and bring your elbows together again in front of you, lifting your head and stretching your neck up, clasping the sides of your neck with your palms. Repeat 5 times. This is an excellent exercise for cervical spondylosis sufferers, since pain in this condition can spread to the shoulders, back of neck, arms and shoulder joints. All of these areas are stimulated gently to increase blood flow, while holding the back of the neck prevents you from stretching too far back.

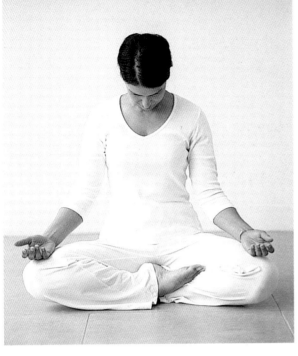

Neck Lock
Jalandhara Bandha

1 Sit comfortably, holding your spine, neck and head straight. Place your hands on your knees and take a deep breath in. While holding your breath, press your chin down into your chest, or as low as is comfortable without pushing it down. Hold for 5 seconds initially, working up to 10 seconds. Breathe out slowly and lift your head, straightening your neck and relaxing your shoulders.

Fish Pose II

Matsyasana

This is a modification of the Fish Pose, which is safer and very effective for most patients in lengthening the neck and spine.

1 Lie on your back with your knees up and your feet on the floor, your arms by your sides. Breathe in deeply as in Ujjayi breathing and lift your spine off the floor up to the nape of your neck. Push your chest up, press your shoulder blades together on the floor and keep your neck straight.

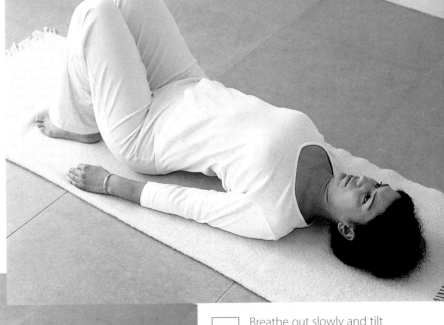

2 Breathe out slowly and tilt the pelvis to roll the entire spine slowly back down onto the floor. The neck will automatically straighten in this position. Repeat 10 times.

The Triangle

Trikonasana

This posture stretches more of the shoulders and neck, releasing upper back tension. Avoid it if your neck is stiff or if you suffer from sciatica as it would be too big a stretch and may cause strain. Only perform this posture when any neck pain has subsided.

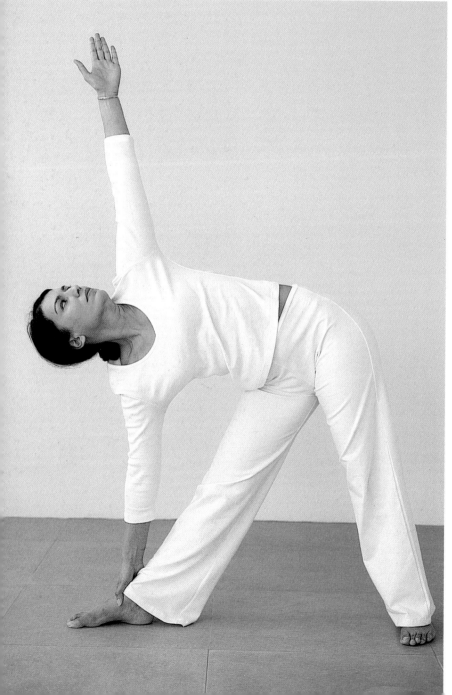

1 Stand with your feet 1–1.5 metres apart. Swivel your right foot out by 90° and turn the left one inwards slightly. Slowly lower your right hand towards your right leg and raise the left arm up with your palm facing forward. Keep your wrist in line with the front of your shoulder.

2 Bend sideways as far as you can, sliding your right hand down your leg. You will feel a gentle stretch on the right side of the back. Hold the position and breathe in and out for 5 seconds, looking up at your left hand. Inhaling, slowly come up and stretch your arms out at shoulder level. Change feet positions, exhale and lower your body towards your left foot. Repeat 5 times on each side. Over time, you may place your right hand in front of the right foot. This gives more of a stretch to the front of the left shoulder.

3 When you've finished, relax in Child's Pose (see page 62) for at least a minute.

backache

Your spine is supposed to be the 'central axis' of the body, much like the trunk of a tree or the weight-bearing axis of a tower. However, all of your organs – your heart, lungs, intestines, liver, spleen and so on – are in front of your spine and there is nothing at the back to counterbalance the weight of these organs. Your spinal muscles therefore have to work extremely hard to keep your back straight and prevent you from falling flat on your face. These muscles also create an anti-gravitational force that keeps your spine erect.

Unlike most other muscles in your body, which contract to facilitate movement, the spinal muscles actually extend. Postural muscles, deep within the spinal muscles, extend the spine and decompress the intervertebral discs (sacs of a gelatinous substance that lie between the vertebrae and act as shock-absorbers). Backache is often blamed on these discs, but in fact the primary cause of back pain is a weakening of the upward thrust created by the postural muscles.

Excess body weight, weak muscles, lack of muscle tone, fatigue, stress, nutritional imbalance and inflammatory disease (such as rheumatoid arthritis) can all weaken the spinal muscles, triggering a concertina effect which causes the discs to compress. When this occurs, the discs can press on a spinal nerve, causing excruciating pain, loss of feeling and tingling. The discs may also bulge or rupture when compressed.

Walking, swimming and yoga are the best exercises for posture control and are therefore excellent for maintaining the back. The various asanas or postures in yoga rely heavily on the spine, so the spinal muscles are exercised thoroughly. Moreover, yoga asanas are performed with breathing techniques that help to provide your muscles with optimum oxygen. A good supply of oxygen to the muscles helps to eliminate inflammation of the tendons – the tissue that attaches your muscles to your bones – and remove lactic acid (a by-product of intensive exercise or activity). Because most backaches are caused by inflammation of the tendons and a build-up of lactic acid, yoga can help to cure backache.

diet The collagen in your ligaments is affected by acidic foods, causing them to weaken. Try to reduce or eliminate citrus fruits (lemons, oranges and grapefruits), pineapple, tomatoes and also spicy foods from your diet, and cut out white wine and champagne. Replace them with plenty of fresh fruits (provided they are not citrus fruits), protein in the form of eggs, fish and chicken to help build up your muscles, potassium-rich foods such as carrots, to tone your muscles, and calcium to strengthen your bones. Make sure you are getting lots of vitamins and minerals. Avoid excess alcohol, which dehydrates your muscles, coffee and salt as these substances cause

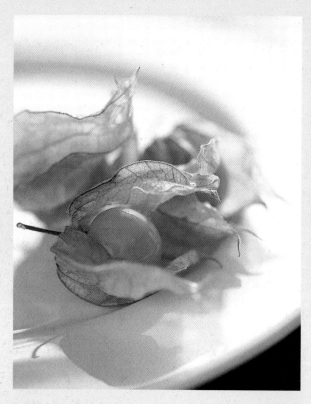

your muscles to tense up, and smoking, which impairs blood flow to your muscles, causing cramps. Eat slowly to improve your digestion, and either have a light dinner or take a walk after a more substantial one to activate the digestive process.

massage Because of the inaccessibility of the back, self-massage is difficult. But a partner massage is very effective, so enjoy one whenever the opportunity arises. If you are giving a back massage, you are likely to come across sore spots on the spinal muscles and tendons. These are due to a build-up of lactic acid and inflammation of the tendons caused by repetitive strain. By rubbing these spots with the ball of your palms or your thumb, you will get more fresh blood (and therefore oxygen) into the muscles and the ache will gradually go away. If you can, mix up a special Back massage oil with 100 ml sesame oil, 1 ml clove oil and 2 ml mustard.

Massage the entire spine, starting at the base and working right up to the tendons of the neck muscles attached to the base of the skull. Use your thumbs or fingers to make firm, circular motions. After loosening the spinal muscles, massage the gluteal region (the buttocks) and the hamstring (on the back of the thigh) as these take a lot of strain while sitting or standing. Altogether this back massage should take 10–15 minutes.

We have discovered, after years of experience, that a painful, twisted back may well be caused by very low-level pain in the groin area, which results in a misalignment of the lower back. If the back is slightly twisted to one side, find a sore area in the groin in the same side. It will probably be just above the pubic bone. Massage this area with your fingers, gently at first and then firmly. This will correct the lop-sided posture and bring fast pain relief.

Therapeutic postures

The following sequence gently stretches out the postural muscles, disperses any lactic acid that has accumulated in the spinal muscles, exercises the tendons and activates the muscles that help to maintain an upright posture.

Embryo Pose I
Pavanmukhtasana

1 Lie on your back. Breathe in and bring your right knee to your chest, pulling the knee towards you.

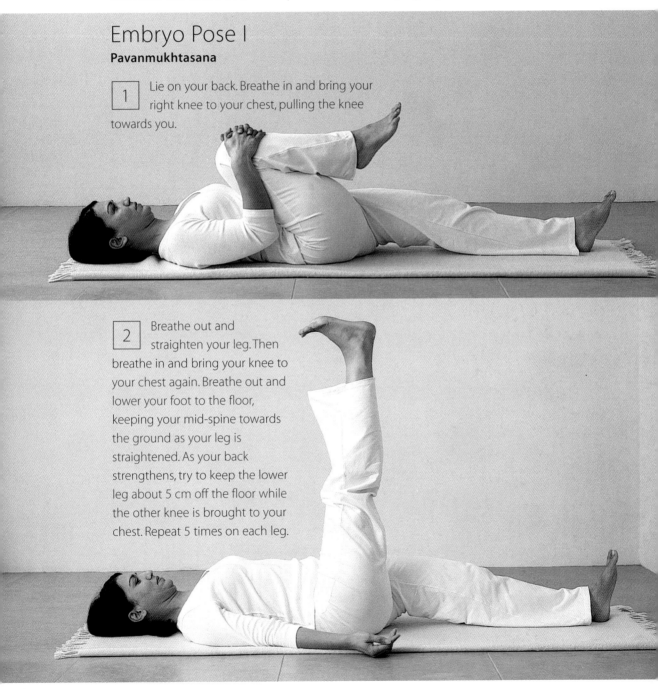

2 Breathe out and straighten your leg. Then breathe in and bring your knee to your chest again. Breathe out and lower your foot to the floor, keeping your mid-spine towards the ground as your leg is straightened. As your back strengthens, try to keep the lower leg about 5 cm off the floor while the other knee is brought to your chest. Repeat 5 times on each leg.

Supine Twist II
Supta Parivritasana

1 Lie on your back on the floor with your knees up and your feet together in front of you, and stretch your arms out to the side at shoulder level. Keep your spine firmly pulled towards the floor at this stage. Now raise your feet off the floor.

2 Lower your knees down to the floor on left, with your knees in line with your hips. Keep your neck straight and stay in the position for 4–5 breaths, easing your upper back towards the floor as you slowly breathe out. Now bring your knees up to your chest before lowering them to the other side. Repeat 5 times on each side. Then bring both knees to your chest and hug them to you, keeping your neck straight, as in the Embryo Pose II (see page 96).

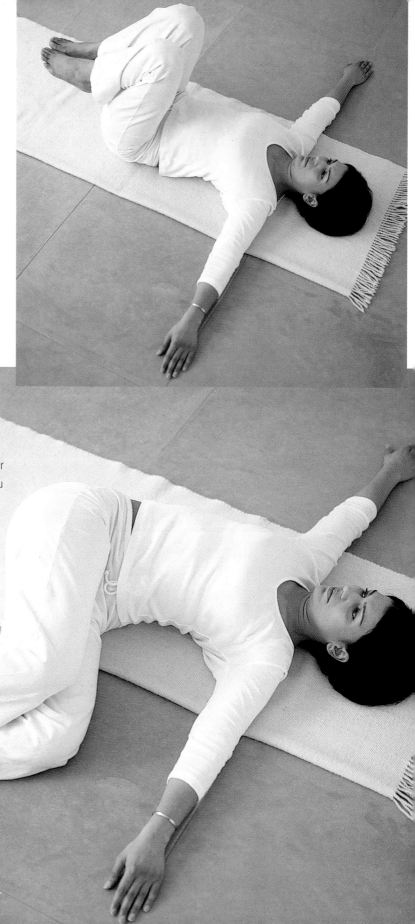

Straight-Leg Lift
Supta Janusirsasana

Move onto these next postures when you have loosened up with the first two poses.

|1| Lie down on your back with your legs straight and slightly apart; make sure your knees haven't turned out. Take a deep breath in and lift your left leg straight up. Breathing out, hold onto your leg and slowly try to reach for your ankle, keeping your head and spine on the floor. If your hamstrings are too tight and you can't reach your ankle with a straight leg, bend your right knee with your right foot flat on the floor.

|2| Breathe in and stretch your arms up over your head, making sure your back doesn't arch off the floor. Breathe out and lower your leg to the ground, keeping the mid-arch of the spine comfortably towards the floor. Repeat 2 or 3 times on each leg.

|3| Repeat Steps 1 and 2, this time lifting your head and shoulders off the floor. Gradually you want to touch your head to your knee – but don't strain! Breathe normally. This helps to correct flat backs and high hips.

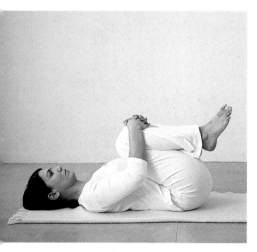

Embryo Pose II
Pavanmukhtasana

1 Lie on your back with your arms by your sides, your shoulders relaxed towards the floor and your neck straight. Breathe in, using Ujjayi breathing, and lift up both knees to your chest. Make sure your back doesn't arch off the floor.

2 Breathe out and lower your feet to the floor again, keeping the mid-arch of your spine comfortably towards the floor by pushing your ribcage down towards your hips. Repeat 10 times. If this exercise is painful, return to the one-legged version on page 93 until your back is strong enough to perform this two-legged variation.

Hero's Pose
Virasana
This exercise strengthens your legs and hips, and is good for correcting forward-leaning posture.

1 From a standing position, take a long step forward with your right foot and bend the knee; bend your other knee slightly, too. Now bend your right arm as shown. Breathe in and straighten your right arm, thrusting it forward. Then breathe out as you step forward with your left leg and repeat on this side. Keep stepping forwards in this way, 10 times on each side. Try to stay in the pose a little longer as you gain in strength.

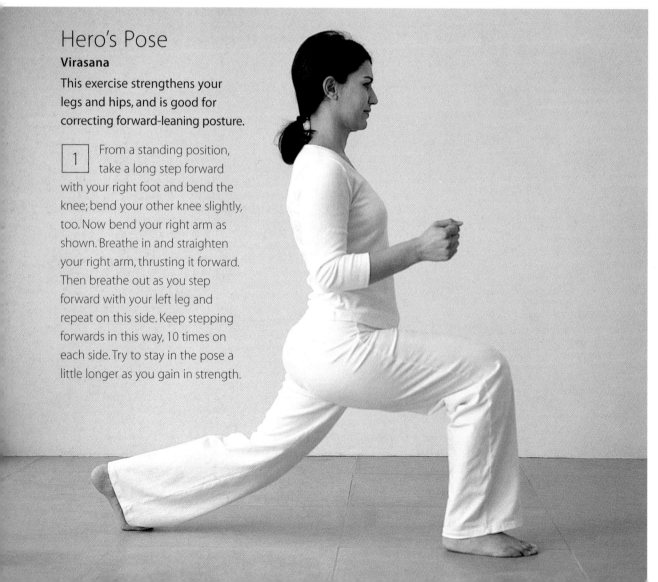

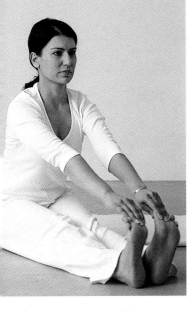

Forward Stretch Paschimottanasana

When you can comfortably hold this posture without feeling a stretch, your spine is at a healthy level of vertebra and disc separation. You can do any other form of exercise as long as you can achieve this level of stretch. If not, cut out the exercise and resume more stretching. This will ensure the health of your discs forever. Progress carefully to this level, however, without strain.

1 Sit up straight with both legs stretched out in front of you and inhale deeply. Hold your toes and straighten your back and neck. Stay in the stretch for 4–6 breaths, working up to 12 breaths, maintaining a constant rhythm in your breath. Then sit back slowly, keeping your shoulders down and back. Try to lift your spine up on sitting back, to help keep your lower back free of tension.

The Locust II Shalabasana

This posture is particularly good for relieving sciatica.

1 Lie on your stomach with your arms by your sides and your chin on the floor. Inhale and lift your left leg straight up, keeping the front of your hips on the floor. Exhale and lower it slowly to the floor. Over time, hold for an extra breath before lowering the leg. Repeat 5 times on each side.

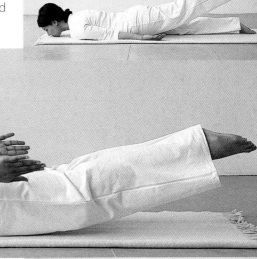

2 Gradually, as your back strengthens, lift both legs and arms off the floor and look up. Repeat 5 times. If your back is strong enough to hold the position for longer, perform just one repetition.

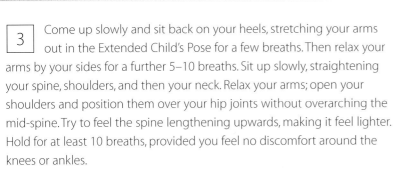

3 Come up slowly and sit back on your heels, stretching your arms out in the Extended Child's Pose for a few breaths. Then relax your arms by your sides for a further 5–10 breaths. Sit up slowly, straightening your spine, shoulders, and then your neck. Relax your arms; open your shoulders and position them over your hip joints without overarching the mid-spine. Try to feel the spine lengthening upwards, making it feel lighter. Hold for at least 10 breaths, provided you feel no discomfort around the knees or ankles.

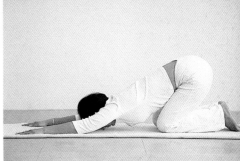

The Cobra **Bhujangasana**

This improves the backward extension of your spine, which is as much a function of a healthy spine as the forward bend. If you can stay in full Cobra (Step 3) without any pressure on the lower back, your back is tension-free bending backwards.

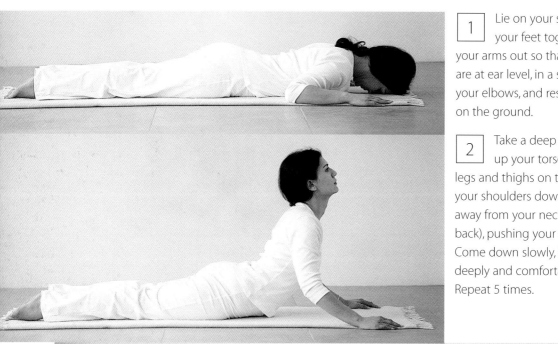

1 Lie on your stomach with your feet together. Spread your arms out so that your hands are at ear level, in a straight line with your elbows, and rest your forehead on the ground.

2 Take a deep breath in and lift up your torso, keeping your legs and thighs on the floor. Press your shoulders down and back, away from your neck. Look up (not back), pushing your chest forwards. Come down slowly, breathing as deeply and comfortably as possible. Repeat 5 times.

3 Over time, move into the full Cobra by straightening your arms, and work up to holding the pose for 12 breaths. Breathe out and lower your forehead back to the floor.

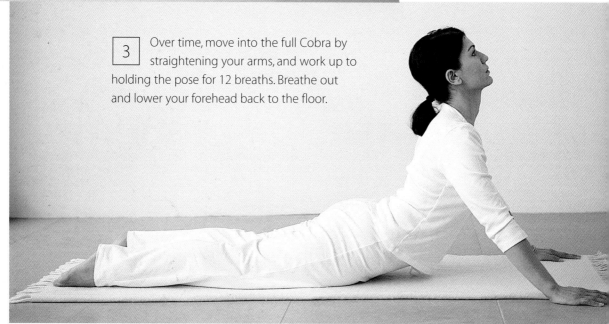

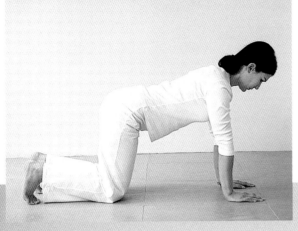

Downward Dog

Adho Mukha Svanasana

If you have rounded shoulders or feel hunched in the back, this posture can help to stretch you out again.

1. Kneel on all fours and curl your toes under your feet.

2. Lift your knees off the floor, straighten your legs and stretch your heels towards the floor. Try and lock out your arms (otherwise the pressure on the joints would be too great) and stretch down your head and back. Keep your spine straight and relax your neck, letting it stretch away from your shoulders. Hold for 4–5 breaths.

3. At the end, arch your spine down and let go of the neck, allowing it to stretch away from your shoulders for 5 breaths or so. Slowly straighten your neck, keeping the arch of your spine stable.

4. Come down slowly onto your knees and relax in the Child's Pose (see page 62).

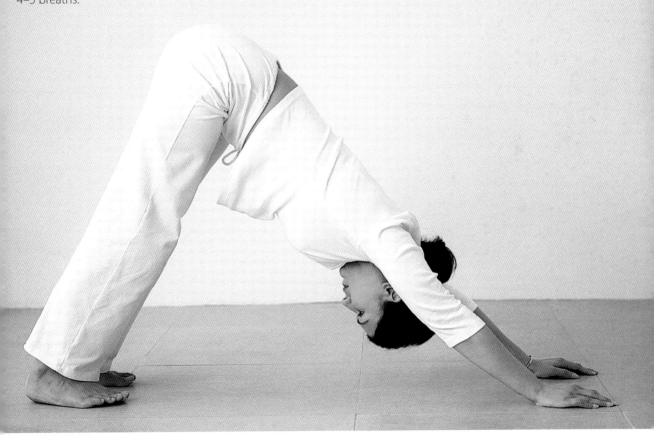

Cross-Legged Pose

Siddhasana

Once your back is strengthened, you may attempt to sit in the Cross-Legged Pose, which helps to straighten your spine. It is one of the most comfortable postures for the back and is easily attainable by most people. The triangular base provides increased stability for the rod-like spine. Try to lift the entire back upwards without accentuating the mid-spine arch.

1 Sit on the floor, initially with your back against a wall, and cross your legs. Place your hands on your knees with your palms up or down. The palms-up position can help to lift a heavy mind, which prevents the back from sinking too heavily into the floor. The palms-down position will help to ground you if you feel light-headed or are drifting off.

2 Finish the session by lying in the Corpse Pose (see pages 46–47) for at least 10 minutes.

repetitive strain injury

Keyboard operators, musicians, machinists, decorators, athletes and manual labourers often use the same muscles over and over again without a break in the course of their work. These muscles then get so overworked that they start to develop a number of symptoms including pain, tingling, inflammation swelling, cramps and knots in the muscles (due to the build-up of lactic acid), numbness, weakness and often loss of function. This is known as repetitive strain injury or RSI. The hands, wrists, arms, shoulders and neck are most often affected, although the legs and feet can also be vulnerable. RSI is a progressive condition, tending to get steadily worse if it's not treated early enough.

Thanks to the rise in the use of computers, RSI is becoming increasingly widespread. Sitting still for prolonged periods in front of a monitor causes the muscles in the neck to tighten and go into spasm, and a kind of 'rusting' can set in, causing stiffness, pain and often extreme discomfort. What's more, it can limit the flow of blood to the brain and impair the circulation of cerebrospinal fluid, leading to headaches, dizziness, blurred vision, and other unpleasant symptoms. Meanwhile, repeated strokes on the keyboard and mouse movements can damage the muscles, tendons and nerves of the hands, arms and shoulder.

Prevention is the best policy, so you should take steps to ensure that your posture and technique are good, and that your work station is set up as ergonomically as possible. Frequent breaks are also important. If you do start to develop symptoms of RSI, seek treatment straight away to prevent the condition from deteriorating. Massage and exercises are very effective at strengthening the muscles.

diet Avoid all acid foods, as excess acid delays the healing process. Excess salt and coffee cause you to tense up your muscles, which can exacerbate the symptoms of RSI. Drink alcohol in moderation, if at all.

massage A couple of times a week, preferably at bedtime, massage your neck and

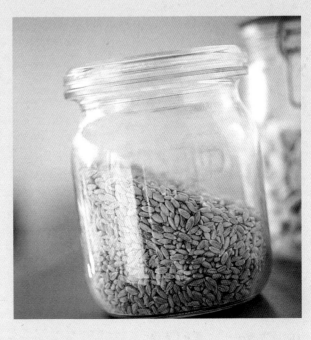

shoulders, as well as your arms and hands, with Dr Ali's Muscle Fatigue and Pain Oil (add 1 ml each of clove and ginger oil and 0.5 ml each of menthol and wintergreen oil to 100 ml sesame oil). During a bath or shower, soak your neck and shoulders for a couple of minutes and massage them to break down any lactic acid and improve blood flow to these vulnerable areas.

An arm and hand self-massage can help to relieve the pain of RSI. Grasp your elbow with your thumb and fingers and slide your hand down to your wrist, massaging the muscles on the outside of your lower arm. Then rotate your arm and repeat the same movements on the inside of your forearm. Next locate the tendon of the biceps muscle (usually a tender cord descending from the shoulder to the biceps in the front of your arm) and keep massaging it down to the bulk of the biceps until the pain eases. Finally, use your thumb to massage the palm and fingers of your other hand.

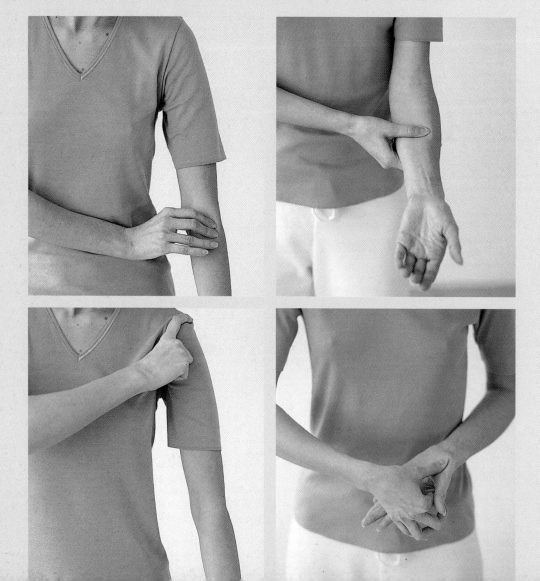

Therapeutic postures

These exercises are aimed at reducing tension in the shoulder joints, which frees up your arms and relaxes your neck.

Swinging Tree
Hastottanasana

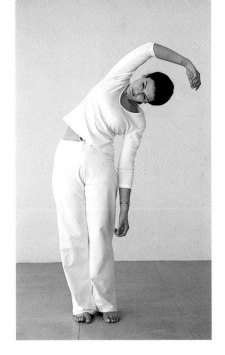

1. Standing with your feet slightly apart, breathe in and raise your right arm above your head. Stretch to your left without moving your hips, and relax your neck. Breathe out and come up to the centre again. Now breathe in and repeat on the other side. Complete 5–10 stretches on each side.

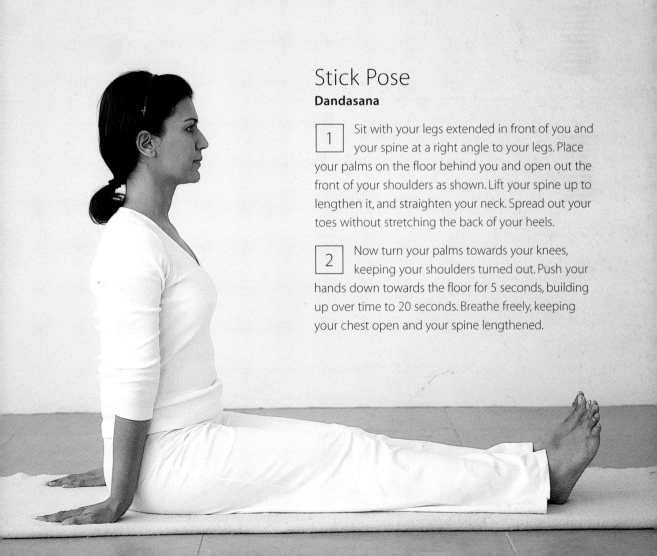

Stick Pose
Dandasana

1. Sit with your legs extended in front of you and your spine at a right angle to your legs. Place your palms on the floor behind you and open out the front of your shoulders as shown. Lift your spine up to lengthen it, and straighten your neck. Spread out your toes without stretching the back of your heels.

2. Now turn your palms towards your knees, keeping your shoulders turned out. Push your hands down towards the floor for 5 seconds, building up over time to 20 seconds. Breathe freely, keeping your chest open and your spine lengthened.

Eagle Pose
Garudasana

This is an excellent exercise for twisting all the tired muscle attachments around your elbow and wrist joints. Do it as often as you can each day.

1 Intertwine your arms by placing the outside of your right elbow over the outside of your right arm near the elbow. Then enclose your left hand in your right palm. Lower your hands below your eye level as far as you can without hunching your spine. Breathe deeply and comfortably, keeping your chest relaxed. Hold the stretch for 5–10 breaths, then repeat on the other side.

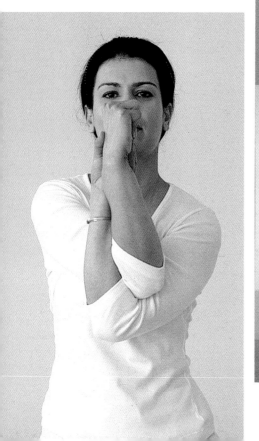

Postural Cycle
Asana Vinyasa

These quick exercises are easy to perform at work and help to keep your spine free of tension, thereby reducing the build-up of repetitive strain in your arm muscles.

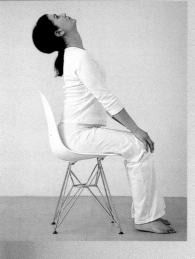

1 Sit on a sturdy chair with your back straight and your hands on your knees. Breathing in, pull your shoulders back, pushing your shoulder blades together, open your chest forwards and slowly look up to stretch the front of your neck and chest.

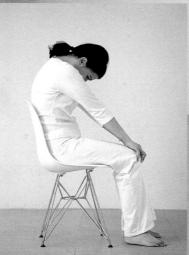

2 Breathing out, slowly lower your head to your chest. Round your back and spread out your shoulder blades, keeping hold of your knees as much as you can. Breathe normally for a few seconds.

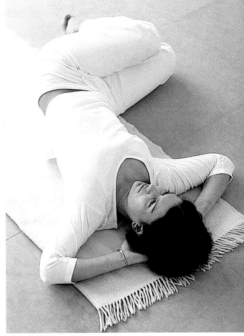

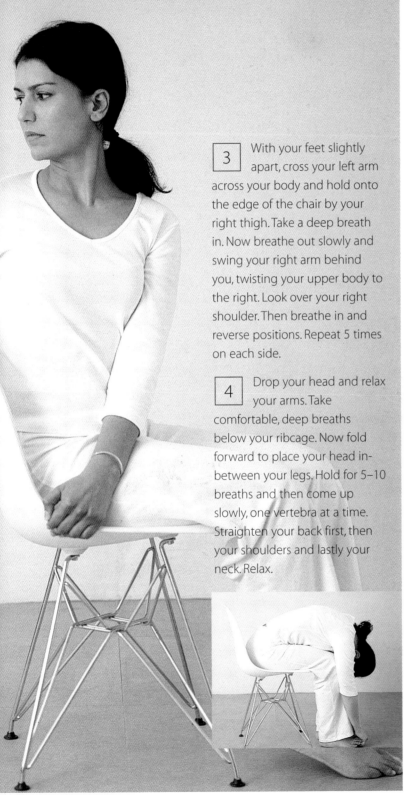

3 With your feet slightly apart, cross your left arm across your body and hold onto the edge of the chair by your right thigh. Take a deep breath in. Now breathe out slowly and swing your right arm behind you, twisting your upper body to the right. Look over your right shoulder. Then breathe in and reverse positions. Repeat 5 times on each side.

4 Drop your head and relax your arms. Take comfortable, deep breaths below your ribcage. Now fold forward to place your head in-between your legs. Hold for 5–10 breaths and then come up slowly, one vertebra at a time. Straighten your back first, then your shoulders and lastly your neck. Relax.

Supine Twist III
Supta Parivritasana

1 Lie on your back with your hands under your head and your feet together on the floor, your knees bent. Relax. If your shoulders are painful, straighten out your arms.

2 Breathe in, lift your knees up to your chest and then lower them towards the floor on the right, at a right angle to your torso. Hold the position for 10–15 breaths and breathe out slowly, relaxing your upper body completely. Repeat to the other side.

3 Straighten out your legs and relax in the Corpse Pose (see pages 46–47). Stretch your neck out by looking alternately over your right and left shoulders.

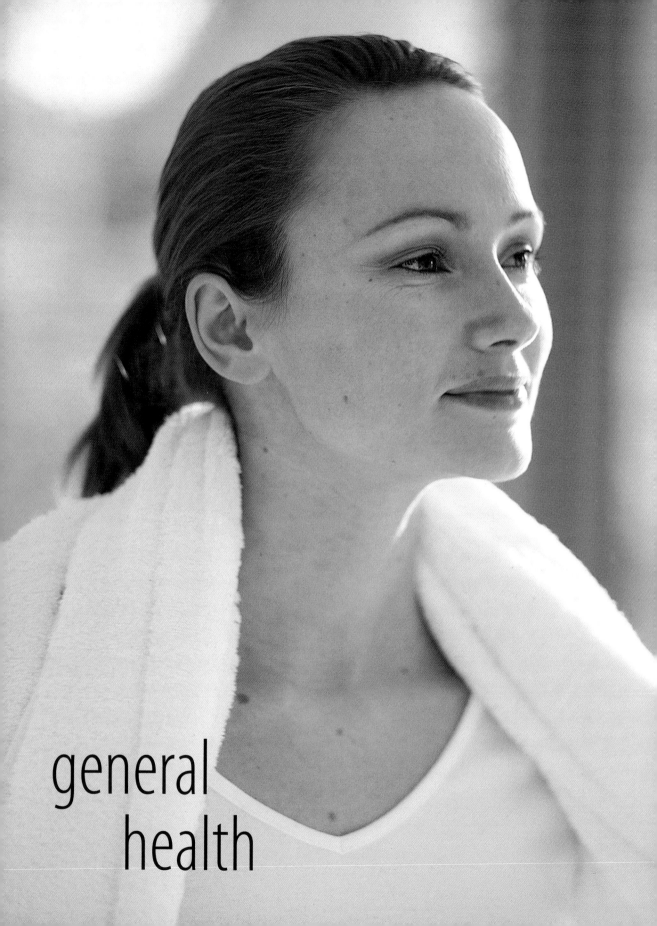

general
health

chronic fatigue syndrome

Also known as ME (myalgic encephalomyelitis), chronic fatigue syndrome, or CFS, is a complex collection of symptoms dominated by extreme, prolonged fatigue. Other symptoms experienced in about 60 per cent of cases include muscle pain, lack of concentration, short-term memory loss, sleep disturbances, depression, headache, a 'muzzy' head, panic attacks, blurred vision, tinnitus, bloating or abdominal gas and hormonal disturbances.

Although glandular fever or another viral infection such as flu or gastroenteritis, seems to be the trigger in about 20 per cent of cases, no definitive cause of CFS has yet been identified. In our view, a number of different factors are probably involved. We have found that poor blood flow through the vertebral arteries in the neck (due to misaligned vertebrae) to the base of the brain is the predominant cause in about 60 per cent of the cases we see. Other factors include: vitamin and mineral deficiencies (particularly of vitamin B_{12}, magnesium, calcium, iron and zinc); chronic sinus problems, which cause congestion and heaviness in the head; clinical depression; low blood pressure; a severe lack of sleep; and poor protein intake.

Because so many factors are likely to trigger the disorder, our approach includes a whole range of therapies that are designed to work together to kick-start the healing process and alleviate the symptoms.

diet Avoid yeast products, sugar, citrus fruits, alcohol, cheese, mushrooms and coffee as these foods disrupt your digestion and may cause the malabsorption of essential nutrients, which will just add to your fatigue. To boost your energy, make sure you eat lots of protein-rich foods such as eggs, fish, chicken, tofu, cottage cheese and soaked almonds; apples, pears, bananas, kiwis and other fresh fruits; plenty of fresh vegetables, which are good sources of vitamins and minerals; and a daily glass of carrot juice.

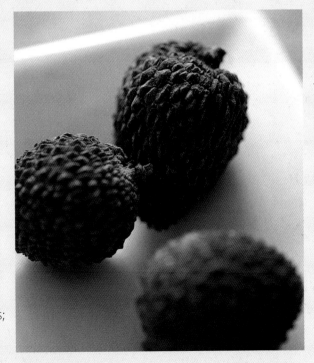

nutritional treatment Although you cannot administer this yourself, sometimes a cocktail of vitamins and minerals, injected into your bloodstream, can help to kick-start the body. A physician with experience in this area should be consulted. He or she will select the vitamins and minerals most appropriate for each case; vitamins C and B_{12} and the minerals magnesium, calcium and selenium are often prescribed. For those who have developed chronic fatigue syndrome following glandular fever, these injections and oral supplements are particularly helpful as the virus that causes glandular fever attacks the mitochondria, or power stations, within the cells, particularly in the muscles, causing massive power failure all over the body and making the muscles inert and painful.

massage Regular deep tissue massage of the neck and spine area followed by monthly adjustment of the upper spine by a qualified, experienced chiropractor or osteopath, is highly recommended for anyone suffering from CFS. But a self-massage can also be very effective. You'll need to press quite hard, using your fingers to disperse any knots and sore points in the tissue. Starting at the base of your skull, work along your neck to the top of your shoulders. Then use circular movements with your fingers or thumbs to massage your jaws and temples.

training at an altitude

Over the past 12 years, we have conducted numerous health trips to the Indian Himalayas. At a comfortable altitude of 1500–1800 metres, patients undertake a residential programme of diet, therapeutic yoga, graded walks for 3–4 hours daily and remedial massage. The effect of this programme on CFS is almost miraculous. Patients become energetic and most of their symptoms disappear within days. After a prolonged period of fatigue and depression, the change in environment combined with careful therapy brings about phenomenal changes in the mind and body.

How does the programme work? The thin air at high altitude invigorates the body's blood-producing system, boosting haemoglobin levels and increasing the body's oxygen supply. At the same time, the therapeutic yoga and massage invigorate the mind and body, helping the body to adapt to the altitude. The more patients walk, the more their confidence builds. At the end of the two-week stay, patients are advised to continue their exercise plan back home by walking in the countryside and going to the gym or swimming. This helps to maintain their newfound good health.

Therapeutic postures

Therapeutic yoga can help to eliminate the symptoms of CFS and restore wellbeing. It has two main effects on the body. First, it increases blood flow to the parts of the brain that control mental and emotional health, thus helping to tackle symptoms such as depression, sleep disturbances, lethargy, panic attacks and lack of concentration; it also activates the pituitary gland, which secretes feel-good chemicals called endorphins. And second, the postures combined with a focus on breathing increase the blood supply to the muscles (removing lactic acid and reducing muscle ache) and the various organs, improving physical wellbeing. Yoga is therefore a great regime for rehabilitating the body following CFS.

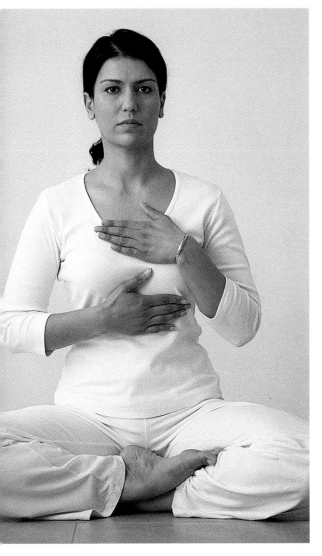

Complete Breath
Ujjayi Pranayama

Most people with CFS have developed poor breathing habits; as their bodies weaken, so do their breathing mechanisms. A deep breath often creates immediate dizziness as they do not have a normal level of oxygen in their bloodstreams. So, developing better breathing habits is very important in their course of treatment.

1 Sit in a comfortable position (or lie down if you are new to yoga). Take a deep Ujjayi breath without force. Hold your breath for 5 seconds. Increase this gradually to 10 seconds.

2 Raise your ribs and contract the pubis and anus to lift them upwards; this is known as an Anal Lock or Mula Bandha. You may now feel a little tension in your head. To counterbalance this, lower your chin to your sternum in a Chin Lock or Jalandhara Bandha, which should help to relieve the tension. Try to feel every inch of your lungs and skin filling up with air, keeping your face, neck and arms completely relaxed. Breathe out slowly, relaxing both locks. Resume normal breathing for a few seconds and then practise the Complete Breath again. Repeat 10 times, then lie down in the Corpse Pose (see pages 46–47).

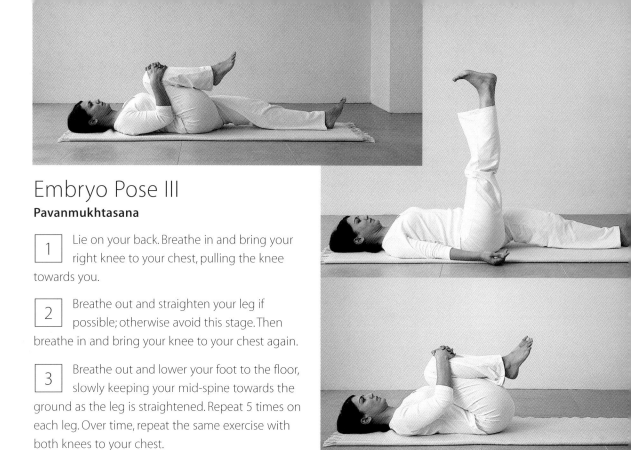

Embryo Pose III
Pavanmukhtasana

| 1 | Lie on your back. Breathe in and bring your right knee to your chest, pulling the knee towards you. |

| 2 | Breathe out and straighten your leg if possible; otherwise avoid this stage. Then breathe in and bring your knee to your chest again. |

| 3 | Breathe out and lower your foot to the floor, slowly keeping your mid-spine towards the ground as the leg is straightened. Repeat 5 times on each leg. Over time, repeat the same exercise with both knees to your chest. |

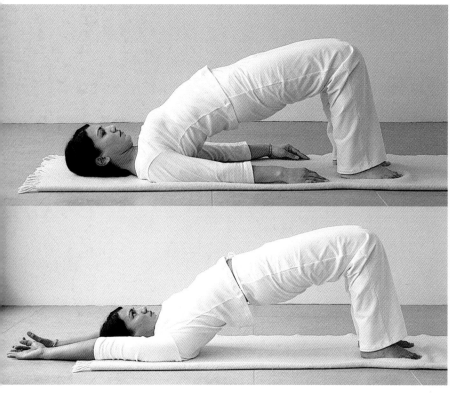

The Bridge
Setubandhasana

| 1 | Lie on your back with your arms by your sides, your knees bent and your ankles below your knees, hip-distance apart. Breathe in and peel your back off the floor until just your head, shoulders and feet are in contact with the floor. Keep stretching your neck while your back is lifted. Come down slowly on breathing out. Relax. Repeat 5 times. |

| 2 | Repeat Step 1 but this time raise your arms up over your head, stretching your arms away from your shoulders. |

Supine Twist IV

Supta Parivritasana

This twist is excellent for relieving tension in the upper back. In our experience, this part of the spine is almost always weakened in CFS sufferers, and this exercise helps to straighten and strengthen it.

1 Lie on the floor with your knees up and your feet together in front of you, and stretch your arms out to the side at shoulder level.

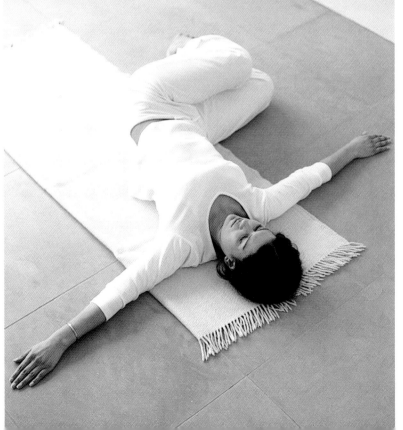

2 Slowly lower your knees to the right, looking over your left shoulder as you do so. Press your right shoulder and upper back towards the floor. Over time, try to increase the distance between your feet until you reach a stage where on lowering the knees towards the right, the left knee is touching the right ankle. Slowly come up, pelvic tilt and repeat on the other side.

3 Repeat Steps 1 and 2, this time raising the knees to your chest and then lowering them so that your knees are in line with your hips. Keep your neck straight and stay on each side for 4–5 breaths, easing the upper back to floor as you slowly breathe out.

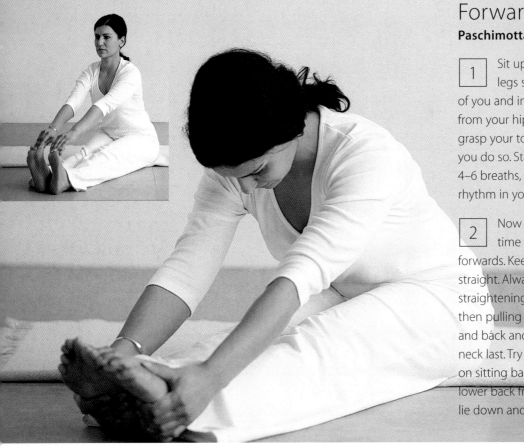

Forward Stretch
Paschimottanasana

1. Sit up straight with both legs stretched out in front of you and inhale deeply. Bending from your hips, reach forward and grasp your toes, slowly exhaling as you do so. Stay in the stretch for 4–6 breaths, keeping a constant rhythm in your breath.

2. Now repeat Step 1, this time folding further forwards. Keep your upper back straight. Always sit back slowly, straightening your spine first, then pulling the shoulders down and back and straightening the neck last. Try to lift your spine up on sitting back, to help keep your lower back free of tension. Now lie down and breathe normally.

Straight-Leg Lift
Supta Janusirsasana
If you are very stiff, you may not be able to do the Forward Stretch without rounding your upper back. If this is the case, try these Leg Lifts first.

1. Lie down on your back with your legs stretched out. Lift your right leg straight up, keeping your spine pulled in towards the floor, and hold on to your calf or ankle. Hold for 4–6 breaths. Lower the leg slowly. Repeat twice with each leg.

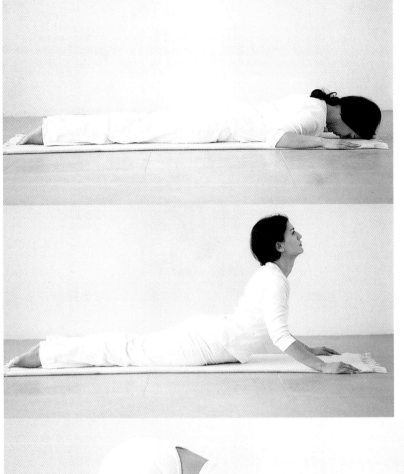

The Cobra
Bhujangasana

1. Lie on your stomach with your feet together. Place your hands at ear-level, your elbows against the floor, and rest your forehead on the ground.

2. Take a deep breath in and lift up your torso, keeping your legs and thighs on the floor. Press your shoulders down and back, away from your neck. Look up (not back), pushing your chest forwards. Breathe out and lower your forehead back to the floor. Repeat 5 times. If your arms tire, lift up your upper torso without putting pressure on your hands.

3. Rest in the Extended Child's Pose, with your arms stretched out in front of you, for 12 breaths.

4. Slowly drag your arms back to sit back on your heels, keeping your forehead on the floor and relaxing your arms in the Child's Pose (see page 62).

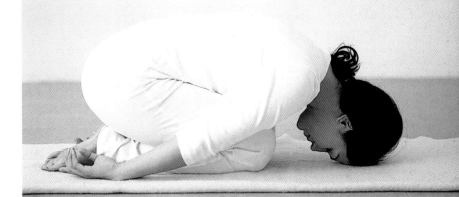

Headstand
Sirsasana

1 Start in the Child's Pose with your elbows by the sides of your knees.

2 Take a deep breath in and slowly come up on your knees to roll onto the crown of your head, taking most of the pressure onto your hands. Hold and breathe out. Remain in the pose for 4–5 comfortable breaths and relax your facial muscles.

3 At the end, breathe in, then breathe out slowly as you sit back in the Child's Pose. Resume normal breathing and stay in this position for at least 1 minute. Slowly sit up and completely relax your arms, straightening your back first without arching it, then your shoulders and lastly your neck.

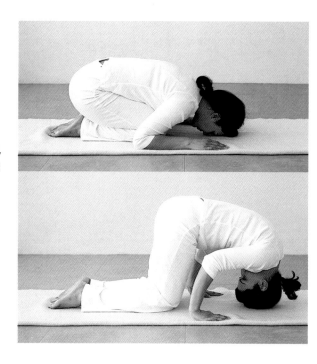

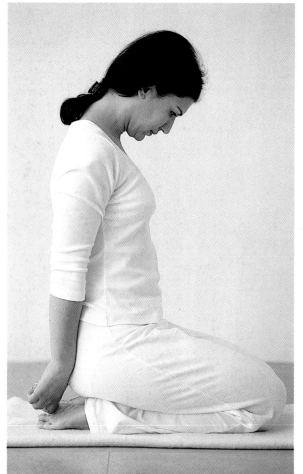

Blessed Posture
Bhadrasana

This pose is hugely beneficial as it gently stretches out the vertebral column and neck, as well as opening the lungs. Fixing your gaze on the tip of your nose will help you still and calm your mind and hence develop concentration.

1 Continuing to sit on your heels, bring your feet together under your buttocks and grasp hold of your right toe with your right hand and your left toe with your left hand. Lower your chin to your sternum and gaze at the tip of your nose for 10–12 breaths. Relax your breath, making it slow and even.

2 Release the pose and place your left hand in your lap, palm up. Using your right hand to close your nostrils, perform 5 cycles of Alternate Nostril Breathing (see page 34).

headaches and migraines

Most people experience a headache from time to time. This common medical complaint can be felt as a dull, throbbing ache or sharp, shooting pains, and may spread across the whole head or be concentrated in one particular area. Migraine headaches tend to be more severe, and are usually accompanied by other symptoms such as nausea and photophobia (sensitivity to light).

Fortunately, the causes of most headaches lie outside the brain, which is very well protected by the skull, the fluid around the brain and the blood–brain barrier (a special membrane which filters out most chemicals in the blood other than oxygen, glucose, a few drugs and alcohol, so that only selective substances reach the brain cells). The majority of headaches originate in the neck: about 60 per cent occur when blood flow in the vertebral arteries in the neck is restricted due to misalignment of the spine. Other causes include sinus problems, tension, insomnia, changes in blood sugar level or blood pressure, tension in the jaw, infections, food intolerance, anaemia, dehydration, certain drugs, excess alcohol and smoking.

Treating a headache with painkillers may help to relieve the pain, but it will not tackle the underlying problem; it is far better to eliminate the cause itself. Because so many headaches originate in the neck, yoga and therapeutic massage play an essential role in preventing and curing such headaches.

A migraine is a collection of symptoms that occurs periodically – weekly, monthly or even yearly. One of the main symptoms is a severe headache, usually one sided (the word migraine comes from 'hemi' or half and 'crania' or head). Migraines are often accompanied by what is known as an aura (early symptoms that appear before the onset of the severe headache), nausea, vomiting, sensitivity to light and sound, anxiety and extreme fatigue. Attacks often last for more than a day. Women are more prone to migraines than men, and often experience an attack 2–3 days before menstruation.

Although powerful painkillers and other medications may help to suppress a migraine headache, drugs will have little or no effect on the actual progress of the condition. Some drugs, like betablockers, simply mask the symptoms. Our experience shows that the Healthy Living Routine (pages 24–47), with a strong emphasis on therapeutic yoga and massage, is most the effective way of dealing with a migraine. A neck massage followed by therapeutic yoga will bring welcome relief during an attack and, over a period of 3 to 6 months, should reduce the intensity and duration of the migraines. Moreover, the cycle of the headaches will become longer and thus they will become more infrequent. If you can predict the onset of your migraines, follow the healthy living routine strictly from a week before the expected attack, and be sure to drink plenty of water.

During an acute migraine attack, practise retention breathing. Inhale for 3 seconds, hold your breath for 6 seconds and then exhale for 6–9 seconds. This builds up the level of carbon dioxide in your blood, which helps to dilate your blood vessels and hence improve blood flow to your brain as well as saturate your blood with more oxygen.

diet   Certain foods are thought to trigger headaches in some people, so it is worth keeping a food diary to establish whether there are any foods that have this effect on you. It is best to avoid coffee, sugar, chocolate and cakes, excess alcohol, very spicy food, too much salt, dairy products such as cheese, and canned products, as these can all bring on a headache. Above all, keep hydrated: make sure you drink 6–8 glasses of water every day. Biorelaxation Tea, containing peppermint and rose, is also useful as it relaxes your muscles and induces calm.

massage   Self-massage can be very effective for relieving a headache, particularly if you catch it before it really takes hold. Starting at the base of your skull just above the hairline, massage downwards to the top of your shoulders. Using your thumb and fingers, rub these areas intensively until they become relatively pain-free. Then, with the help of your fingers, massage your jaw joint for a couple of minutes. Next, work on the temples and the area at the lateral end of your eyebrows.

If you are one of the many headache sufferers who experiences pain at the base of your skull where the tendons of your neck muscles are attached, you may find it soothing to lie on your back with a hot water bottle against the side of your neck. Move it to the other side after 3 minutes.

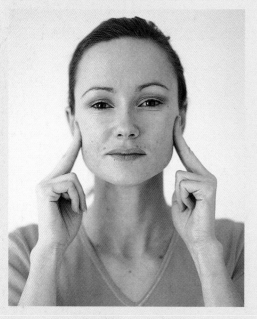
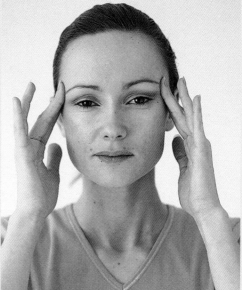

Therapeutic postures

Stretching and strengthening the upper back to release the pressure from weak or tightened ligaments at the base of the skull is crucial in the treatment of headaches, as is proper relaxation. Start off with the exercises for backaches (pages 93–100) for a few weeks. Once your back has strengthened, add the following postures to further build up your upper spine. In all the postures, try to coordinate the movements with your breath, using either Ujjayi or Abdominal Breathing (page 33).

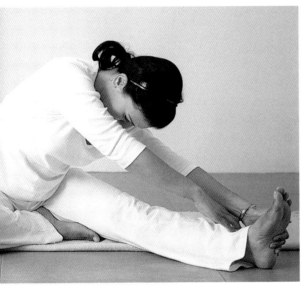

One-Legged Forward Bend
Janusirsasana

This stretches your arms, the back of your shoulders, your hips and upper back as well as your legs. It provides a wonderful de-tenser for all the muscles around the hip and shoulder joints.

1 Sit with both legs stretched out in front of you, your back straight. Bend your right leg so that the heel is against the left thigh. Stretch forwards towards your left foot with your hand towards the outside of the left ankle. Stay in the stretch for 4–5 breaths. Always sit back slowly, straightening the spine so that it feels buoyant when upright. Repeat 2–3 times on each side.

The Bridge
Setubandhasana

1 Lie on your back with your arms by your sides, your knees bent and your ankles below your knees, hip-distance apart.

2 Grasp hold of your ankles, breathe in and peel your back off the floor, starting at the hips, until just your head, shoulders and feet are in contact with the floor. Don't strain. Keep stretching your neck while your back is lifted. Come down slowly on breathing out. Repeat 5 times.

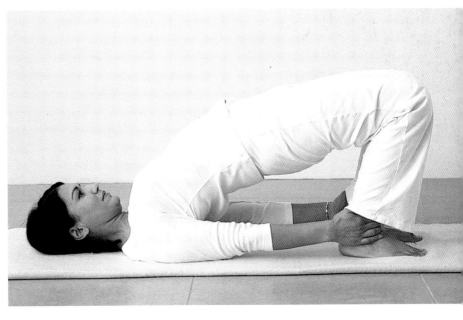

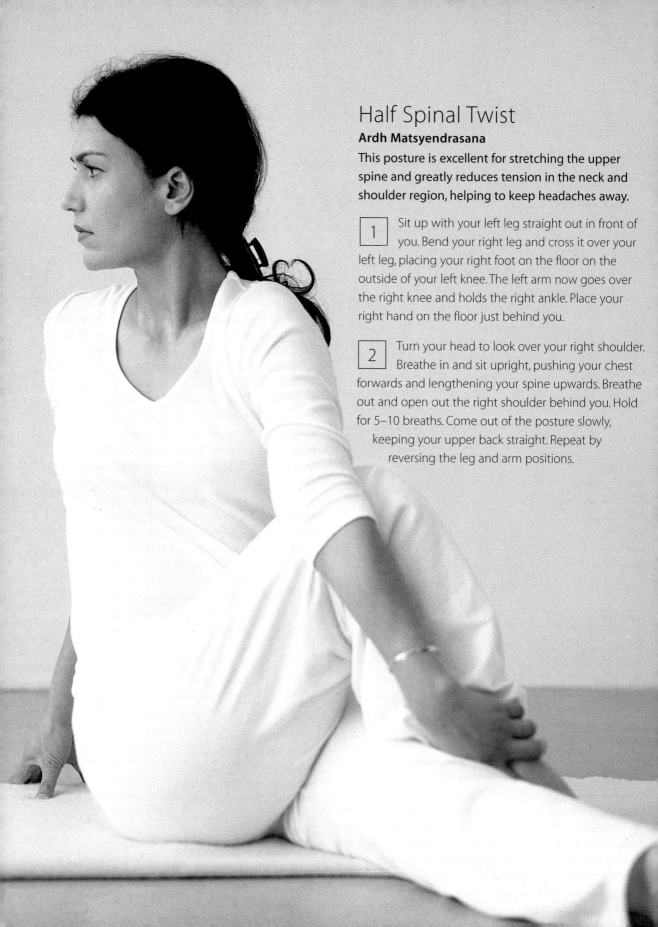

Half Spinal Twist

Ardh Matsyendrasana

This posture is excellent for stretching the upper spine and greatly reduces tension in the neck and shoulder region, helping to keep headaches away.

1 Sit up with your left leg straight out in front of you. Bend your right leg and cross it over your left leg, placing your right foot on the floor on the outside of your left knee. The left arm now goes over the right knee and holds the right ankle. Place your right hand on the floor just behind you.

2 Turn your head to look over your right shoulder. Breathe in and sit upright, pushing your chest forwards and lengthening your spine upwards. Breathe out and open out the right shoulder behind you. Hold for 5–10 breaths. Come out of the posture slowly, keeping your upper back straight. Repeat by reversing the leg and arm positions.

Forward Stretch
Paschimottanasana

1 Sit up straight with both legs stretched out in front, and inhale deeply. Bending from your hips, fold forward as far as you can, slowly exhaling as you do so. Hold for 5–10 breaths. Sit up slowly, straightening your spine first, pulling your shoulders down, and then straightening your neck.

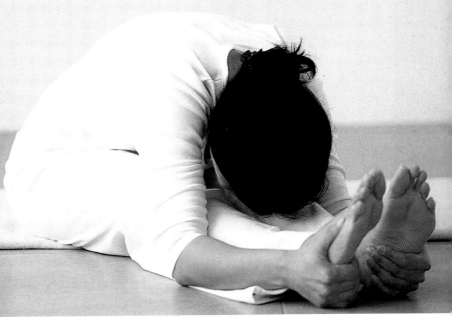

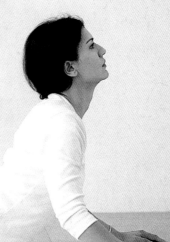

The Cobra
Bhujangasana

1 Lie on your stomach with your feet together. Place your forehead and forearms on the floor, with your hands at ear level.

2 Take a deep breath in and lift up your torso, keeping your legs and thighs on the floor. Press your shoulders down and back, away from your neck. Look up (not back), pushing your chest forwards. Breathe out and lower your forehead back to the floor. Repeat 5 times. Over time you may stay in the posture for 5 breaths and do it just once when you no longer feel the pressure on your lower back. Rest in Child's Pose (see page 62), then repeat 10 cycles of Alternate Nostril Breathing (see page 34).

Corpse Pose

Shavasana

1 Lie down on your back, with your feet apart and relaxing outwards, your arms a little away from your body, palms up. Take a deep breath in and stretch the back of your neck away from your shoulders by lowering your chin towards your chest. Breathe out slowly and let go of your neck and shoulders, allowing them to 'sink' towards the floor.

2 Turn your head to the right so that your right ear touches the floor. If your left shoulder rises up from the floor, keep pulling it down. Hold for 2–3 breaths. Then let go of the arms and neck but remain in this position. Relax your breathing and your whole body, including your jaw and facial muscles, for 5 minutes. Repeat on the other side. Straighten the neck once more and relax for at least for 5 minutes.

3 Try to retain your breath after inhaling while you are in Corpse Pose. Start by holding it for 5 seconds, and slowly increase to 10 seconds, adding 1–2 seconds at a time. Relax in-between breaths, but make sure you practise 5–10 retention breaths. This allows more oxygen to be absorbed by your tissues and thereby creates deeper relaxation. This is quite an advanced practice, so don't push yourself beyond your capabilities.

insomnia, depression and panic attacks

Sleep is an essential part of life, and a lack of it causes fatigue, saps concentration and above all impairs daytime performance. Insomnia is a chronic inability to fall or stay asleep. Medically speaking, an insomniac is someone who sleeps for less than 3 hours a night, 3–4 times a week or more.

During sleep, a network of nerve fibres in an area of the brain known as the sleep centre, blocks the impulses heading towards the brain surface from the other parts of your body. This frees the conscious brain from stimulation from the rest of the body, allowing you to rest deeply and thoroughly. Like all nerve centres, the sleep centre will function best with a proper flow of blood, which delivers essential fuel in the form of oxygen and glucose. A neck massage and yoga will help to get the blood flowing through the vertebral arteries in the neck and thus aid sleep, particularly if they are done at bedtime. These techniques will also improve the circulation of cerebrospinal fluid in the brain, which in turn will help to supply more glucose and some oxygen to the pineal gland, a small structure in the brain that secretes melatonin – the hormone that slows down metabolism and induces sleep. So massage and yoga, combined with general stretching, relaxation techniques and meditation, are often all you'll need to get a good night's sleep.

Depression is the mental equivalent of chronic fatigue syndrome (see pages 107–108). Whereas CFS sufferers feel physically low, those with depression feel emotionally low: anxiety, pessimism, lethargy and insomnia are all common symptoms. In many cases these feelings lift spontaneously after a few days or weeks, but in some people the depression can be more severe. Interestingly, scientists found that a decreased blood supply to the brain was common to both conditions. The primary aim of any treatment for depression should therefore be to increase the flow of blood to the brain – and massage and yoga do just this. You might find it difficult at first to motivate yourself to follow the yoga plan set out over the following pages, but you will find it a bit easier each time as you start to feel the benefits of greater energy and a calmer disposition.

Shallow breathing, restricted to the upper chest instead of proper diaphragmatic breathing, often accompanies depression, and postural problems can result from holding the diaphragm and related muscles in this limited way. Most people simply get used to a low level of energy or feeling depressed. So when you start to practise yogic breathing and your diaphragm is allowed to move freely, you may experience the surfacing of blocked emotions. These will gradually lessen in intensity and bring about a release of physical and emotional waste products. Breathing freely is one of the simplest ways to strengthen your nervous system and shake off despair.

A *panic attack* is an extreme state of anxiety. Stress causes the neck muscles to go into spasm and decreases the circulation of cerebrospinal fluid, as well as obstructing blood flow through the vertebral arteries that supply blood to the brain. When the areas of the brain that control your breathing and heart beat receive less blood than they should, they put the body into panic mode. So your heart rate goes up, causing palpitations, and you start to breathe more rapidly to increase blood flow to the brain, which can result in hyperventilation. The best way to control a panic attack is to hold your breath. This raises the amount of carbon dioxide in your blood and improves the possibility of oxygen exchange in the lungs, which returns your body to its normal physiological state. Breathing into a paper bag until symptoms subside has the same effect.

diet If you have low blood pressure, which causes chronic fatigue and depression, a high protein diet consisting of fish, poultry, eggs and soaked almonds is recommended to normalise your blood pressure. Carrot and apple juice, caviar, marrow bone soup (see page 66), honey and ginger tea have beneficial effects on low blood pressure, too. We also recommend that you take supplements of St John's Wort, which acts as a natural antidepressant, the minerals magnesium and calcium to tone up your blood pressure, and vitamins C and B-complex, which strengthen your immune system and therefore make you better able to cope.

massage The crucial point here is to get blood flowing to the brain, so try to massage your neck and shoulders (or, better still, get someone to massage them for you) as regularly as possible. For advice on how to perform a deep tissue massage on your neck, turn to page 29. This technique also improves the function of the limbic system in the brain, which is primarily responsible for your emotions.

meditation If you have trouble sleeping, or are prone to panic attacks, meditation may be just what you need to calm your mind and induce sleep. Meditation is a deeper, more subtle form of stress relief than other relaxation techniques and numerous studies on transcendental meditation have shown its effectiveness in treating insomnia. For advice on how to meditate, turn to pages 20–21. You may not be able to concentrate for very long to begin with, particularly if you are feeling anxious and find it difficult to still your mind, but with practise this period of relaxed concentration will increase. Remember that whatever you wish for or crave is already there inside you: you simply need to explore and touch it.

Therapeutic postures

A stiff upper back and restricted breathing have been shown to correlate with depression and anxiety. The following sequence of postures stretches the spine to improve blood flow to the brain and facilitates better breathing. This encourages the release of endorphins (the body's feelgood chemicals) from the pituitary gland.

Supine Twist V
Supta Parivritasana

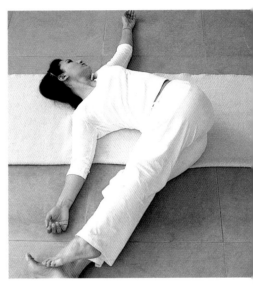

1 Lie on your back with your arms out to the side at shoulder level, palms facing up. Bring both knees towards your chest and then lower them to the floor on the right. Stretch out your legs so that your toes reach towards your right hand. Breathe out and gently look over your left shoulder, feeling the stretch down the left side of your upper back. Hold for 5–12 breaths and then repeat on the other side. On finishing, bring both knees up to the chest for 4–5 breaths.

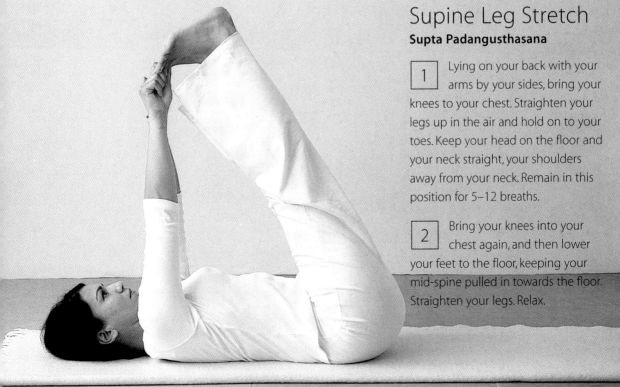

Supine Leg Stretch
Supta Padangusthasana

1 Lying on your back with your arms by your sides, bring your knees to your chest. Straighten your legs up in the air and hold on to your toes. Keep your head on the floor and your neck straight, your shoulders away from your neck. Remain in this position for 5–12 breaths.

2 Bring your knees into your chest again, and then lower your feet to the floor, keeping your mid-spine pulled in towards the floor. Straighten your legs. Relax.

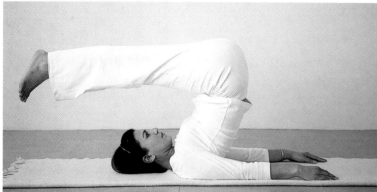

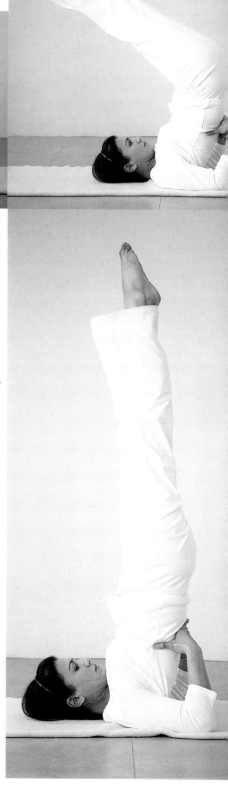

Shoulderstand

Sarvangasana

This is a cleansing as well as a reviving pose. It helps to drain blood from the legs and return it to the right side of the heart and on to the lungs for purification. The reviving effects are brought about by the dilation of the blood vessels in the lungs and the heart. This increases the flow of oxygenated blood to the abdominal organs and the thyroid, thus promoting the proper nutrition of these tissues. The pose is best practised in three stages.

1 Lie on your back with your arms by your sides, your palms facing down. Bend your knees over your abdomen and stretch your legs out horizontally until they form a 90° angle with the floor. Stay in this position for a count of 10–20, your arms relaxed. You may experience a stretch in your hamstrings as your knees straighten; if you can't straighten your legs to 90°, you aren't ready for this posture. Repeat 5 times.

2 From Step 1, try to lift your trunk off the floor, taking the weight of your body onto your arms. Support your back with your hands, your elbows firmly planted on the floor. By sliding your hands lower and lower down your back, you will be able to straighten your spine until it is vertical. Stay for a count of 10, working up to 30 counts with practice.

3 When you can steadily hold position 2, press your chin into the base of your throat without raising your head off the ground. Straighten your legs and tilt them backward until they feel weightless. Hold the pose for 1 minute and work up to a maximum of 3 minutes. Breathe comfortably. Come down slowly, supporting your back with your hands if necessary, straighten your legs and relax.

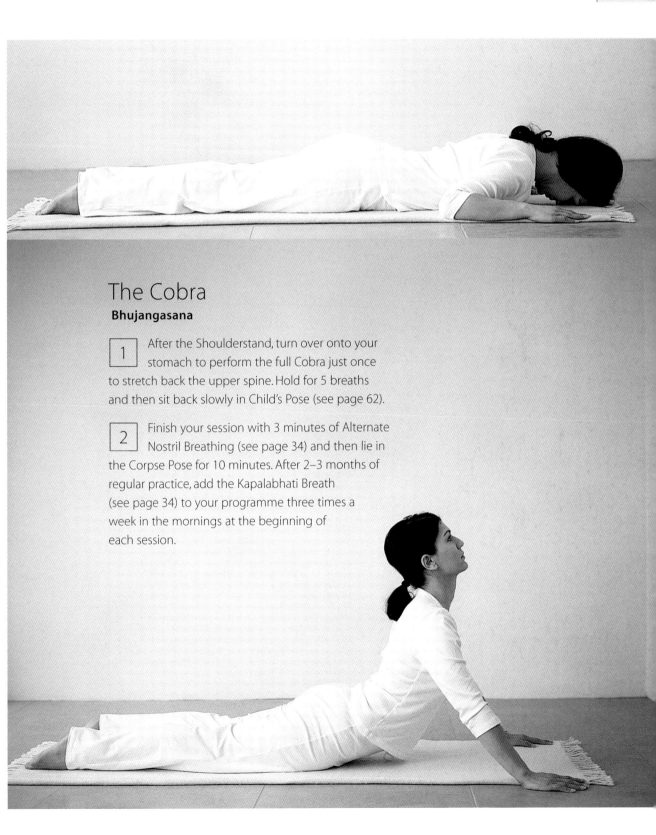

The Cobra
Bhujangasana

| 1 | After the Shoulderstand, turn over onto your stomach to perform the full Cobra just once |

to stretch back the upper spine. Hold for 5 breaths and then sit back slowly in Child's Pose (see page 62).

| 2 | Finish your session with 3 minutes of Alternate Nostril Breathing (see page 34) and then lie in |

the Corpse Pose for 10 minutes. After 2–3 months of regular practice, add the Kapalabhati Breath (see page 34) to your programme three times a week in the mornings at the beginning of each session.

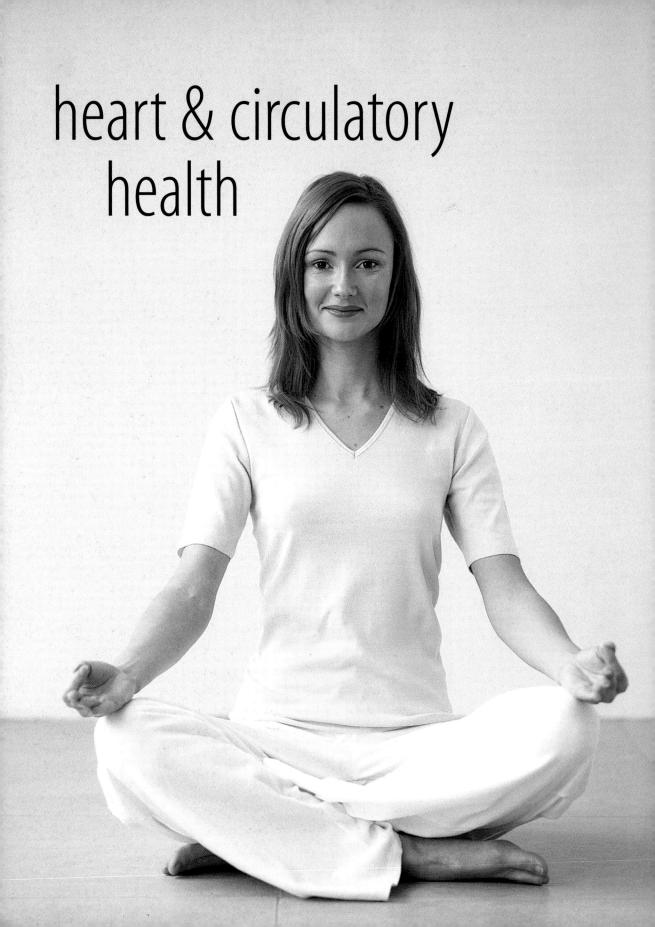

heart & circulatory
health

high blood pressure

Your blood pressure rises and falls naturally throughout the day, depending on how active you are, but when it remains elevated over time, it is known as high blood pressure or hypertension. This common condition of the circulatory or cardiovascular system puts a tremendous strain on the heart as it has to work extra hard to push blood through the body, and can lead to serious health complications such as heart disease, stroke, kidney damage and eye problems.

The heart is a pump that pushes blood around the network of arteries that reaches every corner of your body. The arterial walls have muscles that can dilate and narrow your arteries. When your arteries constrict, blood can't flow through them so easily, and your blood pressure rises. Physical exertion, excitement, tension and other emotional responses increase your heart rate and temporarily raise your blood pressure. Usually it returns to normal once you rest. But in people with hypertension, blood pressure is raised all the time. The causes of high blood pressure may include stress, high levels in the blood of cholesterol (which can clog up the arteries), excess salt or alcohol consumption, smoking, overweight, or another medical condition.

But the truth is that high blood pressure is easy to prevent. We feel that everyone from around the age of 40 onwards – especially if they have a family history of high blood pressure or heart disease – should follow preventative measures. Our prescription consists of a heart-healthy diet, regular massage to relax you and improve your circulation, and yoga, which has the dual benefit of strengthening your body and calming your mind. Several studies have shown that meditation can also help to lower blood pressure by reducing anxiety levels. It is useful for those suffering from angina, too. For more on how to meditate, see pages 20–21.

diet Aim to fast once a week. This doesn't mean cutting food out altogether: simply limit yourself to non-citrus fruits, green salads, vegetable soups, water (try to drink about 1.5–2 litres daily) and herbal teas. Monday is an ideal time to fast as most of us tend to over-indulge at the weekend. Don't be afraid of fasting – it is a very natural thing to do. It gives your body a complete rest and is particularly beneficial for those with high blood pressure as it eliminates your salt intake (too much salt raises blood pressure), reduces weight, calms the mind, removes excess fluid from the body and lowers blood cholesterol levels. Fast once a week for four months, and then twice a month until your blood pressure normalises.

According to yogic principles, you should stick to a vegetarian diet. If you find this difficult to sustain, stick to white meats (chicken without the skin and fat, and turkey) and fish, which will provide all the protein you need.

If you have high cholesterol levels, have been advised by your doctor to lose weight, or there is evidence of heart disease, we recommend the following diet:

• Avoid fats and oils (even olive oil) completely if you have heart disease and or non-hormonal obesity.

• Use garlic, ginger, black pepper and various herbs and spices to flavour your food. When cooking with chillies, use green ones or a small quantity of dry, powdered chilli.

• Steam vegetables and then mix them in a wok with herbs and spices to add flavour, stirring them a little, shortly before serving.

• For white meat dishes, mix herbs and spices – such as coriander, cumin, powdered clove, cinnamon and cardamom – in a little low-fat yoghurt. Marinade the meat in the mixture for a couple of hours if possible, then grill the meat and serve hot. For fish, use dried herbs or spices. Sprinkle the fish with a few drops of lime juice before grilling it.

• Soups are very good in general (provided they are fresh – avoid canned soups). Firstly, you don't need to use any oil or fat. Secondly, they are easy to digest. You can make them thick or wholesome by adding rice; boil it first until it's mushy before cooking it further in the soup. Chicken (without the skin) or fish can be cooked with various vegetables including potato, onions, leeks, courgettes, beans, peas and carrots. Then add flavourings to taste. Use a little magnesium salt if you wish. Cook all the ingredients with the rice for 45 minutes or so, and then serve (blend the ingredients first if you prefer a thick, smooth soup). You can store the soup in the fridge for 24 hours, but after this time it will lose its nutritional value.

• Avoid desserts if at all possible, especially sugary ones. If you do have a dessert, serve it at least an hour after your main meal so that it doesn't interfere with digestion. You can use honey, if necessary, as a sweetener. Fruits, dried fruits and sugar-free jams (containing fructose) are fine in moderation. Dried almonds (soaked for 12–24 hours), pine seeds and walnuts contain less vegetable fats than other nuts and seeds and therefore can be used in desserts.

• You can include low-fat cottage cheese, egg whites (but not egg yolks), low-fat yoghurt and skimmed milk with small amounts of fat in your diet – but avoid full-fat milk products.

massage Your muscles tense up when you are stressed, which increases resistance to the blood flow by squashing the walls of the arteries – all of which pushes up your blood pressure. So a general massage once or twice a week with the Lifestyle Oil (see page 29) will de-stress the body, induce proper sleep and therefore help to normalise your blood pressure. Use sesame oil to massage your entire body at bedtime for 10 minutes and wash the following day.

Therapeutic postures

Sleep is an important factor in treating high blood pressure, simply because it relaxes tensions both physical and mental. The following exercises are all aimed at inducing sleep and reducing your stress levels. Practise just the Corpse Pose for the first month as it brings about a deep relaxation of the muscles which in turn improves circulation in your capillaries. This eases blood flow to the brain without a sudden rush which would send your blood pressure up.

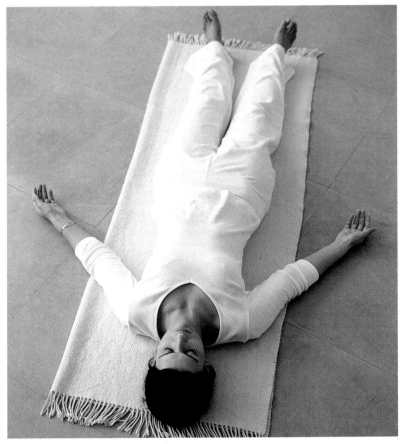

Abdominal Breathing
Pranayama

This is the most natural way to breathe when lying on your back. It relaxes the solar plexus and helps sufficient oxygen to diffuse into the bloodstream without creating tension in your neck and shoulders (which would restrict blood flow to the brain).

1 Lie on your back and relax your arms, legs, head and neck completely. Breathe in through your nose and extend your stomach completely, like a balloon filled with air.

2 Breathe out slowly and let the stomach relax. Do not try to pull your stomach muscles in at this stage. Repeat for at least 20 breaths.

Corpse Pose
Shavasana

1 Lie down on your back with your feet apart and your legs falling gently outwards; keep your arms a little away from your trunk, palms up. Take a deep breath in and stretch the back of your neck away from your shoulders by lowering your chin to the front of your neck. Breathe out slowly and let go of the neck and shoulders, allowing them to 'sink' towards the floor. Relax your facial muscles.

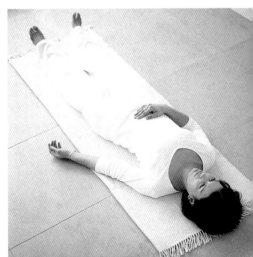

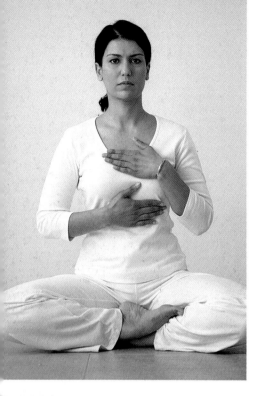

Complete Breath Ujjayi Pranayama

This strengthens the muscles around your heart and increases your lung capacity.

1 Stand or sit cross-legged on the floor. First, breathe out completely. When you inhale, relax your diaphragm (just below your ribcage) and fill up your lungs slowly and steadily by expanding your chest up and out. Remain relaxed and visualise every part of your lungs filling up with air.

2 Now exhale slowly. Try to make your out-breath longer than your in-breath, but stay comfortable. Don't pull in your abdomen – let it relax by itself, so that your lungs remain passive as they empty. Continue for 10 minutes, maintaining the same position and rhythm of breath throughout. If you get a feeling of pressure to the head on breathing in, lower your chin to your sternum, then raise your head slowly on breathing out.

3 When you can perform Steps 1 and 2 without strain or effort, try to start holding your breath for 5 seconds after the out-breaths; increase this over time to 10 seconds. (If you feel flushed or your heart rate goes up, breathe naturally until you are ready to try holding your breath again.) Repeat 20 such breaths.

Supine Twist VI Supta Parivritasana

1 Lie down on your back with your arms out to the sides at shoulder level and your feet together on the floor, your knees bent.

2 Breathe in, lift your knees up to your chest and then lower them towards the floor on the right, at a right angle to your torso. Look over your left shoulder to stretch your neck. Hold the position and breathe out slowly, relaxing your upper body completely. Repeat 5 times on each side.

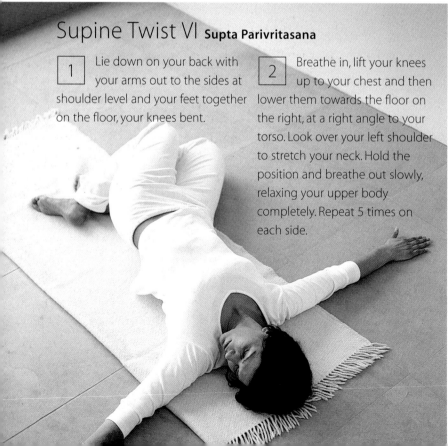

Embryo Pose IV
Pavanmukhtasana

1 Still lying on your back, breathe in and clasp your knees towards your chest for 4–5 breaths. Allow your neck to relax towards the floor and keep the back of your neck long and away from your shoulders.

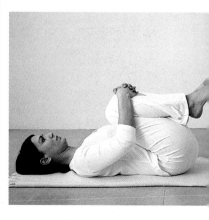

The Bridge
Setubandhasana

| 1 | Lie on your back with your arms by your sides, your knees bent and your ankles below your knees, hip-distance apart.

| 2 | Press your arms along the floor towards your feet and stretch the back of your neck away from your shoulders. Breathe in and peel your back off the floor, starting at the hips, until just your head, shoulders and feet are in contact with the floor. Keep stretching your neck while your back is lifted. Come down slowly on breathing out. Be aware of your alignment: your knees should be the same distance apart on going up and coming down. Repeat 5 times.

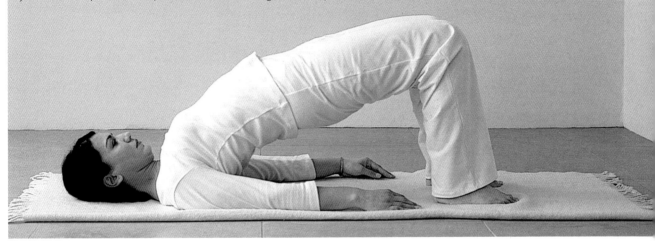

Hamstring Stretch
Urdhva Pavasanta Padasana

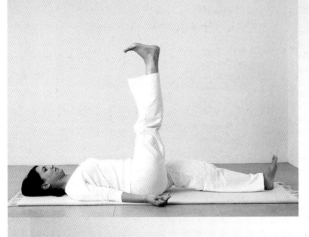

| 1 | Lie on your back with your arms by your sides. Inhale and lift your right leg straight up. Stretch it as far as is comfortable, then lower it slowly to the floor on exhaling, keeping your mid-spine comfortably towards the floor. Repeat 5 times each side.

| 2 | Inhale, expanding your chest, and stretch your arms over your head. Point your toes. Now exhale, relaxing your chest, and lower your arms by your sides. Relax your feet. Repeat 5 times. Then inhale and turn your head to the right so your right ear touches the floor. Keep your left shoulder pressed down. Maintain the stretch on exhaling and then resume normal breathing. Repeat on the other side, then straighten your neck.

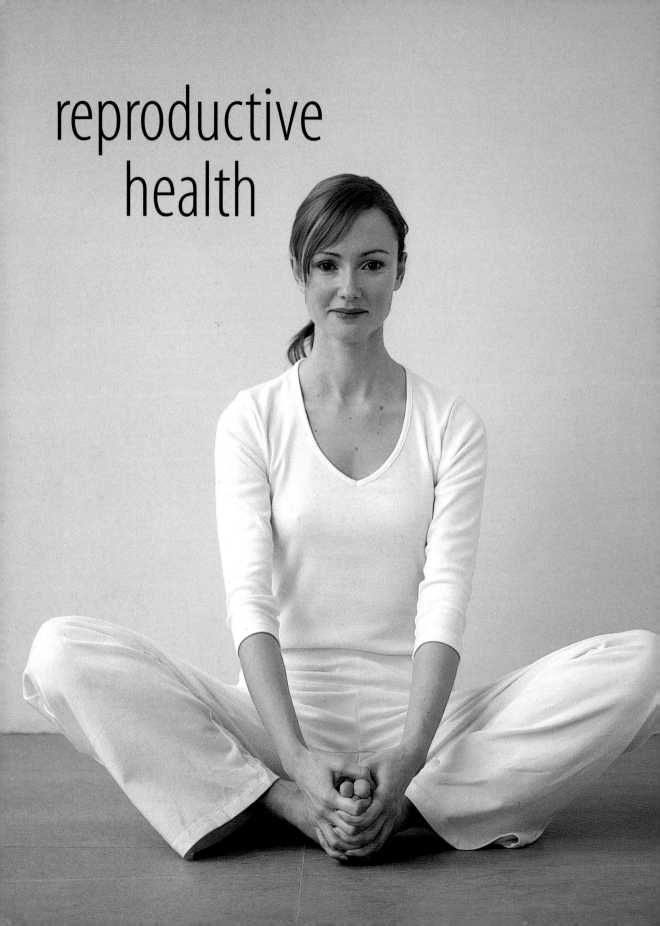

reproductive
health

Menstrual and reproductive issues

All of the major reproductive events in a woman's life – menstruation, pregnancy and menopause – are controlled by hormones, and may be accompanied by certain symptoms. Poor health and stress can adversely affect your hormone levels, so it is essential to keep well and manage your stress levels.

Premenstrual syndrome (PMS) affects many women in the days before menstruation. The symptoms can vary from one individual to another, but the most common include mood swings, lumpy or painful breasts, irritability, bloating, food cravings and headaches. Before the onset of a period, there is massive pelvic congestion as the uterus fills with blood deposits. With so much blood being routed to the pelvic area, the brain receives less oxygen and glucose than usual. As soon as this happens, the range of symptoms known as PMS can appear, especially if the woman has obstructed vertebral arteries due to cervical vertebral misalignment (see page 13), or if she suffers from anaemia or low blood pressure.

Up to 75 per cent of women experience *painful periods or dysmenorrhoea* at some point in their lives. Normally the uterus or womb is suspended by ligaments in a vertical position. If these support ligaments are weak, however, the heavy base of the uterus can tilt forwards or backwards, which causes a kink to form near its opening in the cervix. This kink prevents the blood and cells shed from the uterine lining from passing through, so the uterus begins to contract to push it all out. This is what causes the cramp-like pains. As more blood accumulates, the contractions become increasingly uncomfortable. The pain can last for 2–3 days as the uterus tries to push the blood out without success, and is sometimes so severe that it causes fainting. Finally, after prolonged and severe efforts, the uterus straightens up automatically and pushes the blood out. Almost immediately the contractions stop, bringing instant relief. This is the cause of dysmenorrhoea in the majority of cases, although other conditions, such as fibroids or endometriosis, can also result in menstrual pain.

Pregnancy is a very natural phenomenon, but the body should be well prepared before, well nourished during it, well managed throughout labour and well treated after it. Most women experience a few common complaints at some point during their pregnancies, but these can often be relieved by a combined programme of diet, massage and yoga. During the early stages of pregnancy, get plenty of rest, follow a simple diet (see overleaf) and be sure to relax as much as you can. If you find yourself feeling nauseous, smell green lime. Practice holding your breath, too, to suppress morning sickness: inhale for 3 seconds, hold your breath for 6–9 seconds and then exhale for 6–9 seconds. Yoga is great exercise during pregnancy as it relaxes your body and mind, improves circulation and induces that 'feel-good' factor so important

Great pregnancy poses

Your posture generally is very important during pregnancy. Try to walk without exaggerating the arch in your lower back, and don't turn your feet out. This helps to keep the weight off the front bones of your legs, thereby reducing strain on your spine. Keep your knees slightly bent and lengthen your spine upwards. Release the lower part of your spine by lengthening it and letting it 'drop' down – your pelvis will automatically lift up and position itself below the abdomen. You will also be carrying your baby closer to your spine, which helps to prevent backache. The following exercises are particularly recommended when you are into the fourth month of pregnancy:

- Standing Forward Stretch, page 138
- Cat Pose, page 140
- Downward Dog, page 138
- Cow Pose, page 141
- Tailor Pose, page 141
- Garland Pose, page 139, in the last month
- Pelvic Floor Exercises, page 139
- The Bridge, page 136
- Corpse Pose, page 141

for the healthy development of your baby. During the third trimester, therapeutic yoga is wonderful for toning up your muscles and preventing backache (a common complaint towards the end of pregnancy).

At the end of the reproductive age, the female body goes through some major physiological changes known as the *menopause*. First, periods become irregular, skipping a few months at a time, and often get heavier for a while. This unpredictability causes a lot of stress, especially after years of a rhythmic pattern of periods. For many women, hot flushes are among the worst complications, during which the face suddenly gets flushed, sweating is profuse, the body gets warmer, the heart beats faster and in general there is a feeling of panic. If you experience these flushes, practise holding your breath (as described on page 133) as this helps to alleviate the symptoms. We would advise against taking hormone replacement therapy (HRT) in most cases, unless there is a definite sign of brittle bones. Regular exercise will help you to keep up your bone density and guard against osteoporosis, and combined with healthy eating and stress management, will maintain both your outer and inner beauty.

diet *For PMS*: A week before you expect your period to begin, exclude alcohol, coffee, excess salt, cheese, chocolate, fizzy water, yeast products, canned foods and citrus fruits from your diet.
During pregnancy: Your diet should vary according to the stage of pregnancy. During the first trimester, morning sickness, aversion to food or its smell, and fatigue can

make eating very difficult. At this stage, thick, nutritious soups are very useful, along with soft boiled eggs, puréed vegetables, mashed potatoes, salads and other easily digested foods. Ginger is great for dispelling nausea. Avoid rich, oily, spicy or fried foods and citrus fruits (the acidity can disrupt digestion and cause nausea), which are poorly tolerated, together with alcohol, coffee, excess yeast products (which can cause bloating) and excess sugar. If you can, stick to organic, freshly prepared dishes. Don't worry about your weight during pregnancy: if you don't eat properly you run the risk of not nourishing your baby sufficiently. The time to lose any excess weight will come after the delivery of your baby and when you've finished breastfeeding. When you're breastfeeding, eat plenty of nutritious food with vegetables and fresh, non-citrus fruits and a substantial amount of protein from well-cooked eggs, poultry and fish.

During menopause: Avoid excess salt, coffee and too much alcohol. It's important to keep hydrated, so drink 1.5–2 litres of water a day, and opt for chamomile tea and carrot juice instead of coffee.

massage   *For menstrual cramps:* An abdominal massage can help to relieve pre-menstrual discomfort. See page 54 for details.
During pregnancy: A 10-minute massage of the neck and spine at bedtime is an essential therapeutic tool to boost your wellbeing throughout pregnancy, induce good sleep and reduce anxiety. During the first trimester it can help to eliminate symptoms of nausea and morning sickness. The rapid growth of the embryo means that there is heightened activity in the pelvic region, which deprives the brain of blood – massage can help to get the blood circulating again. Pregnant women should lie on their sides and not their abdomens when receiving a massage: concentrate on the lower back, buttocks, hamstrings and calves.
During menopause: A neck and shoulder massage (see page 29) improves blood flow to the pituitary gland in the brain, which in turn helps to regulate your hormones and relieve hot flushes.

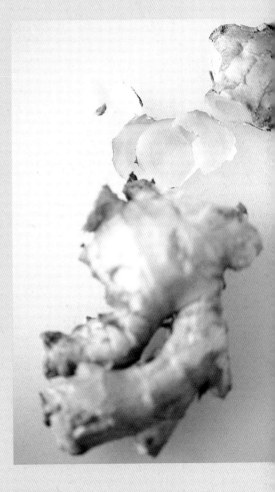

Therapeutic postures

Releasing tension in the pelvic area is crucial in improving circulation in the reproductive organs, and therefore helps to prevent premenstrual symptoms, boost your fertility and ease pregnancy aches and pains. Most of the following stretches and spinal twists are recommended before getting pregnant; you can also follow the yoga sequences suggested on pages 88–90 and 93–100 at this stage. However, avoid spinal or supine twists and cobra during menstruation and if you are pregnant.

Supported Chair Pose
Jangha Sakti Vikasaka

This exercise will help to strengthen your thigh muscles, which is particularly important if you plan on giving birth in an active, squatting position.

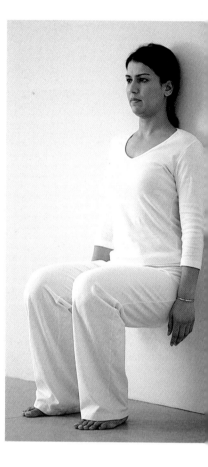

1   Stand against a wall with your feet hip-distance apart, about 30 cm away from the wall. Relax your arms, shoulders and facial muscles and, keeping your feet still, gently slide down the wall as if you were sitting on a chair. Feel your waist against the wall and the lengthening of your lower spine as you slide down. Breathe normally. Repeat twice on a regular basis.

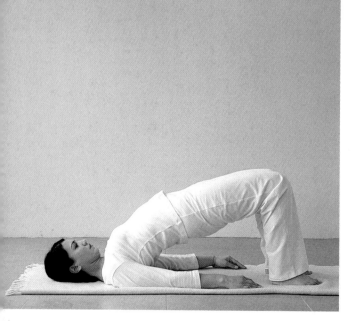

The Bridge   Setubandhasana

1   Lie down on your back to relax the whole spine. Place your arms by your sides and bend your legs so your ankles are beneath your knees, hip-distance apart.

2   Peel your back slowly off the floor, without jolting. Keep your knees above your ankles and push your heels down to the ground. Press down on your hands to steady the posture. Take a deep breath in and stretch your neck away from your shoulders by lowering your chin towards your chest. As you breathe out, slowly lower your back one vertebra at a time, and relax your feet, arms and spine. Repeat twice and then straighten your legs. If your back aches, just breathe in and let your spine rise off the floor naturally; then breathe out and do a pelvic tilt.

Supine Twist VI
Supta Parivritasana

This posture loosens your upper back and reduces strain in the lower back, helping to relieve premenstrual tension. Avoid this exercise, however, if you are menstruating or pregnant.

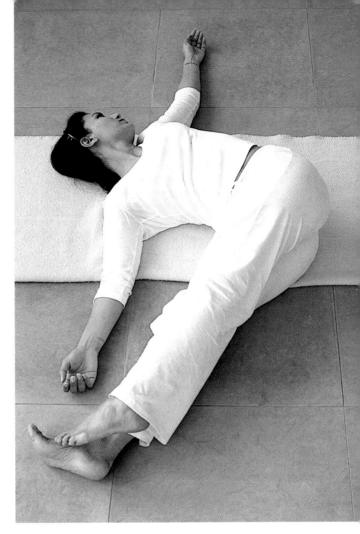

1 Lie on your back with your arms out to the side at shoulder level, palms facing up. Bring both knees towards your chest and then lower them to the floor on the right. Stretch out your legs so that your toes reach towards your right hand. Breathe out and gently look over your left shoulder, feeling the stretch down the left side of your upper back. Hold for 5–10 breaths and then repeat once on the other side. On finishing, bring both knees up to the chest for 4–5 breaths.

2 Finish by breathing in and hugging your knees to your chest in a lying position. Then breathe out and slowly lower your feet to the floor, keeping your spine towards the ground.

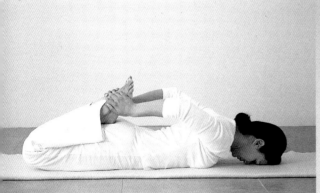

The Bow Dhanurasana

1 Turn over to lie on your stomach, bend your knees and reach behind you to hold onto your ankles. Pull your heels down towards your buttocks, keeping the front of your hips on the floor.

2 Take a deep breath and lift your upper chest off the floor, moving your feet away from your back. Over time, try to lift your knees off the floor as well, and hold for 5 breaths. Don't let your knees move apart. Breathe out and lower your forehead to the floor once more. Repeat 5 times, then sit in Child's Pose (see page 62).

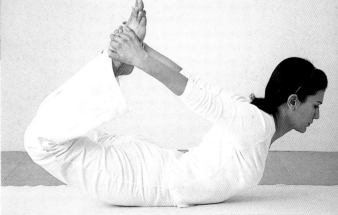

Downward Dog

Adho Mukha Svanasana

This posture can be performed during menstruation as well as before, during and after pregnancy. It brings about a lot of blood to the facial muscles and is an excellent revitaliser from fatigue. It also relaxes the back of the legs, increasing the mobility of the ankles and thereby reducing the likelihood of swollen feet and ankles in later pregnancy.

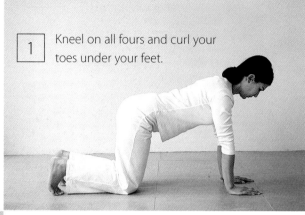

1 Kneel on all fours and curl your toes under your feet.

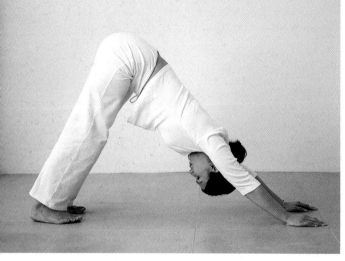

2 Lift your knees off the floor, straighten your legs and stretch your heels towards the floor. Try to lock out the arms (otherwise the pressure on the joints would be too great) and stretch down your head and back. Keep your spine straight and relax your neck, letting it stretch away from your shoulders. Hold for 4–5 breaths.

3 Come down slowly onto your knees and relax in Child's Pose for a few breaths. Then slowly sit up on your heels in Vajrasana or Extended Child's Pose (page 97), relax your shoulders and breathing for a few moments. Try to incorporate periods of relaxation in-between postures during pregnancy.

Standing Forward Stretch

Parvottanasana

This is great for relieving congestion in the pelvic region and can be continued during pregnancy.

1 Stand with your feet apart and then place your right foot about 45 cm in front of your left one. Slowly bend forward so that your back is parallel to the floor, keeping your upper back and neck straight and pulling your chest forwards. Hold for 5 breaths or more, then repeat on the other leg.

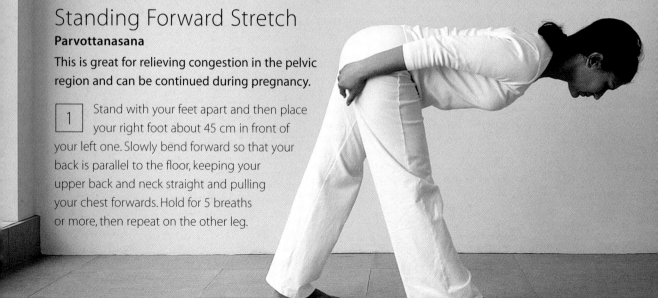

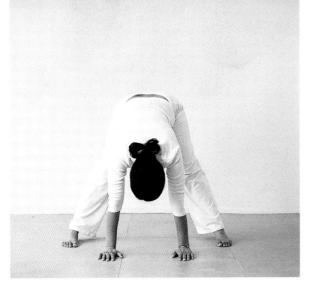

Extended Forward Stretch
Prasarita Padottasana

| 1 | Stand with your feet wide apart. Fold forwards from your hips and place your hands on the floor in front of your feet. Hold for 5–12 breaths. On coming up, bend your knees slightly and roll up your spine, shoulders and neck. Your shoulders, hips and ankles should now be in a straight line. Now move into the Garland Pose. |

Garland Pose **Malasana**

This is excellent for improving the blood supply to the pelvic region and in the last few weeks of pregnancy it can help to manoeuvre the baby's head into the correct position for labour. Omit this exercise, however, if your baby is in a breech position, you have had a cervical suture, or suffer from haemorrhoids or painful varicose veins.

| 1 | To begin with, practise this position by sitting on a stool and pushing your knees open with your elbows; alternatively, hold onto a bar or another person. When you are loose enough, continue without these props, always bending your knees over your toes. Push your palms together in front of your chest and use your elbows to open up your knees and stretch out the hips. Straighten your spine and breathe comfortably. Hold for 12 breaths. |

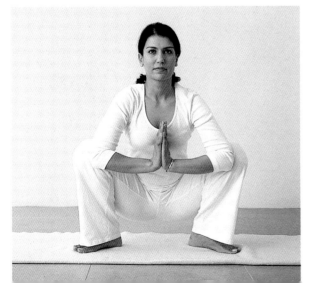

Pelvic Floor Exercises
Mula Bandha

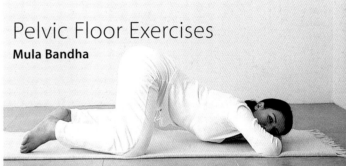

Together with six other ligaments, your pelvic floor muscles support your uterus in the pelvis. These ligaments weaken during pregnancy, so it is important to strengthen them to reduce the risk of backache, miscarriage and stress incontinence. To identify your pelvic floor muscles, imagine clenching the muscles in your pelvic area to stop a flow of urine midstream.

| 1 | Place your knees comfortably apart on the floor and rest your head on your hands. Avoid dropping your mid-spine or letting your abdomen hang down. Breathe in and pull your pelvic floor up towards the uterus. Don't contract your buttocks or abdominal muscles. Breathe out and release slowly. Repeat 10 times. Gradually aim to hold the muscles, breathing out and in once more, before letting go on breathing out. |

| 2 | Repeat Step 1, but this time pull up and release your pelvic floor muscles more slowly, a stage at a time. Breathe normally throughout. Repeat 5 times. |

| 3 | Now pull up and then let go of the muscles rapidly, 10 times in quick succession. Relax and then repeat another 10 times. |

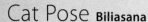

Cat Pose **Biliasana**

This posture safely loosens up the spine and corrects menstrual disorders by releasing the pelvic floor. It is also extremely beneficial for returning the uterus to the correct position after childbirth; you can practise it as either an ante- or a post-natal exercise.

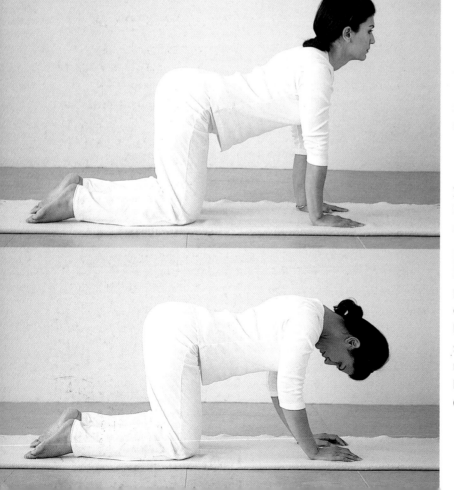

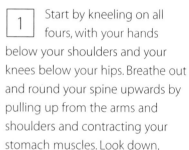

1　Start by kneeling on all fours, with your hands below your shoulders and your knees below your hips. Breathe out and round your spine upwards by pulling up from the arms and shoulders and contracting your stomach muscles. Look down.

2　Breathe in and slowly arch your spine down, pulling your shoulders away from your neck. Stretch your neck forwards, not up. Repeat 5 times.

3　Now arch your spine and relax your head down, pushing your shoulder blades closer together. Feel your neck lengthening away from your shoulders. Hold for 5 breaths, then return to Position 2 on inhaling. Hold and exhale. Finally, sit back in Child's Pose (see page 62).

Cow Pose Gomukhasana

This is an excellent and safe stretch before, during and after pregnancy to lighten the burden on the front of the shoulders and the shoulder blades at the back. Stress in these areas can result from poor posture, heavy breasts or carrying children.

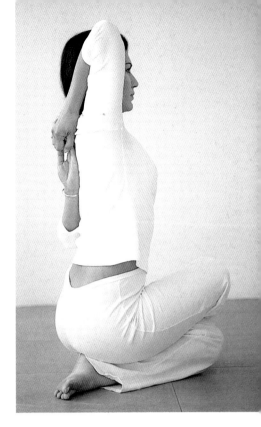

1. Sit on the floor with your legs in front of you. Now bend your left leg so that your heel is under your buttock – in other words, sit on your left heel. Bend your right leg and cross it over your left knee so that both knees are in line, your right heel towards your left hip. (Don't worry if you can't get into this position – sit on a chair or stand instead.)

2. Bend your left arm up behind your back and raise your right arm. Now bend your right arm down at the elbow and try to clasp your hands behind your back. Aim to interlock your fingers over time without forcing the stretch. Remain in the position for 10 breaths. Repeat, reversing positions by sitting on your right heel and lifting up your left arm.

Tailor Pose Baddha Konasana

This posture, also known as the Butterfly Pose, opens out the pelvic area – making it a great exercise to prepare you for childbirth – and increases circulation to the reproductive organs and hips. It also helps to position the pelvis correctly and thus improves posture, but omit this pose if you have chronic back pain.

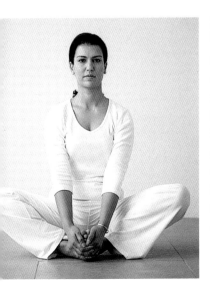

1. Sit on the floor with the soles of your feet together, letting your knees relax down towards the floor. Do not strain or bounce your knees. Holding onto your feet, pull your back straight. Try to lengthen your spine upwards. Sit for as long as is comfortable, aiming gradually to hold the position for 10 minutes. On finishing, straighten your legs out in front of you and relax.

Corpse Pose Shavasana

1. Complete your session by lying in the Corpse Pose (see pages 46–47) and practise slow breathing out. Turn your head to each side 2 or 3 times. If your back aches or arches up too much, bend your knees or lie on your side with one knee bent and placed in front; this position can be practised on its own regularly to stabilise your emotions pre-menstrually, ante- and post-natally.

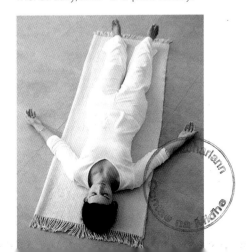

index

acknowledgements

While it is impossible to thank everyone individually who helped us to acquire such in-depth knowledge of yoga, we would particularly like to acknowledge Swami Ram Lakhan, who was a protégé of Dhirendra Brahmhcari, personal yoga therapist to the late Mrs Indira Gandhi. His understanding of yoga in restoring physical and emotional harmony within the body is undoubtedly the best we have come across. Col. B.R. Sharma, who transformed from being a body-builder in his youth to a fine yoga teacher, taught us the various breathing techniques that enable a person to get into various therapeutic postures step by step. Air Vice-Marshall Soren Goyal taught us the philosophy of yoga and its very essence. We would like to thank these and other teachers who helped us to create the foundation of a new but useful approach to yoga – therapeutic yoga.

We would like to thank Grace Cheetham and all her colleagues at Vermilion who helped us through the editing, design and photography.

Finally, we would like to thank the thousands of patients whose practise and feedback on therapeutic yoga helped to put us on the correct path.

We apologise to practitioners of modern-day yoga who may find ours, a very classical and integrated approach, a bit 'out of line' with what they have been taught by their gurus. This is a treatment-based yoga and it had to incorporate diet, massage and other traditional principles of yogic living.

Dr Mosaraf Ali and Jiwan Brar
London 2002

To arrange a medical consultation or to order any of the massage oils mentioned in the book, which are available mail order, please contact:
Integrated Medical Centre
43 New Cavendish Street
London W1G 9TH
Telephone: 020 7224 5111
or visit our website: www.dr-ali.co.uk

For further information on therapeutic yoga classes, please contact:
Yogaworks Ltd
Telephone: 020 7935 9913
or visit our website: www.yogaworks.uk.com

Vermilion would like to thank Sweaty Betty for supplying outfits